THE 30-Day KETO PLAN

THE 30-Day KETO PLAN

Ketogenic Meal Plans to Kick Your Sugar Habit
and Make Your Gut a Fat-Burning Machine

AIMEE ARISTOTELOUS AND RICHARD OLIVA

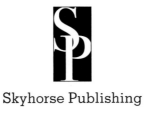

Skyhorse Publishing

Skyhorse Publishing books may be purchased in bulk at special discounts for sales promotion, corporate gifts, fund-raising, or educational purposes. Special editions can also be created to specifications. For details, contact the Special Sales Department, Skyhorse Publishing, 307 West 36th Street, 11th Floor, New York, NY 10018 or info@skyhorsepublishing.com.

Skyhorse® and Skyhorse Publishing® are registered trademarks of Skyhorse Publishing, Inc.®, a Delaware corporation.

Visit our website at www.skyhorsepublishing.com.

10 9 8 7 6 5 4 3 2 1

Library of Congress Cataloging-in-Publication Data

Names: Aristotelous, Aimee, author. | Oliva, Richard, author.
Title: The 30-day keto plan : ketogenic meal plans to kick your sugar habit
    and make your gut a fat burning machine / Aimee Aristotelous & Richard
    Oliva.
Other titles: Thirty-day keto plan
Description: New York : Skyhorse Publishing, [2020] | Includes
    bibliographical references and index. |
    Identifiers: LCCN 2020031235 (print) | LCCN 2020031236 (ebook) | ISBN
    9781510762015 (hardcover) | ISBN 9781510762022 (epub)
Subjects: LCSH: Ketogenic diet. | Reducing diets--Recipes. |
    Low-carbohydrate diet--Recipes.
Classification: LCC RC374.K46 A74 2020 (print) | LCC RC374.K46 (ebook) |
    DDC 641.5/6383--dc23
LC record available at https://lccn.loc.gov/2020031235
LC ebook record available at https://lccn.loc.gov/2020031236

Cover design by Daniel Brount
Cover images from gettyimages

Print ISBN: 978-1-5107-6201-5
Ebook ISBN: 978-1-5107-6202-2

Printed in China

To you, for starting this journey of health, fitness, weight loss, and change.

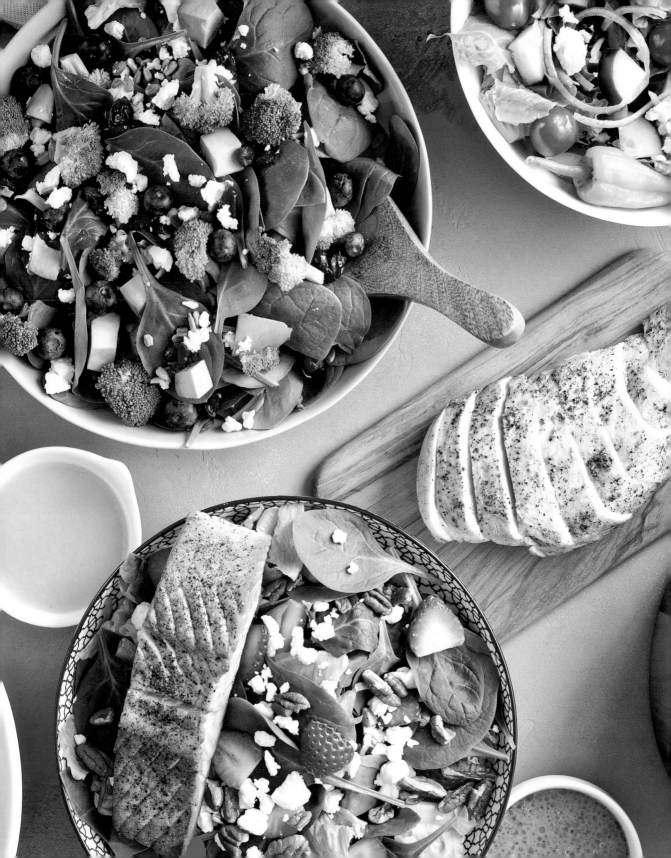

Contents

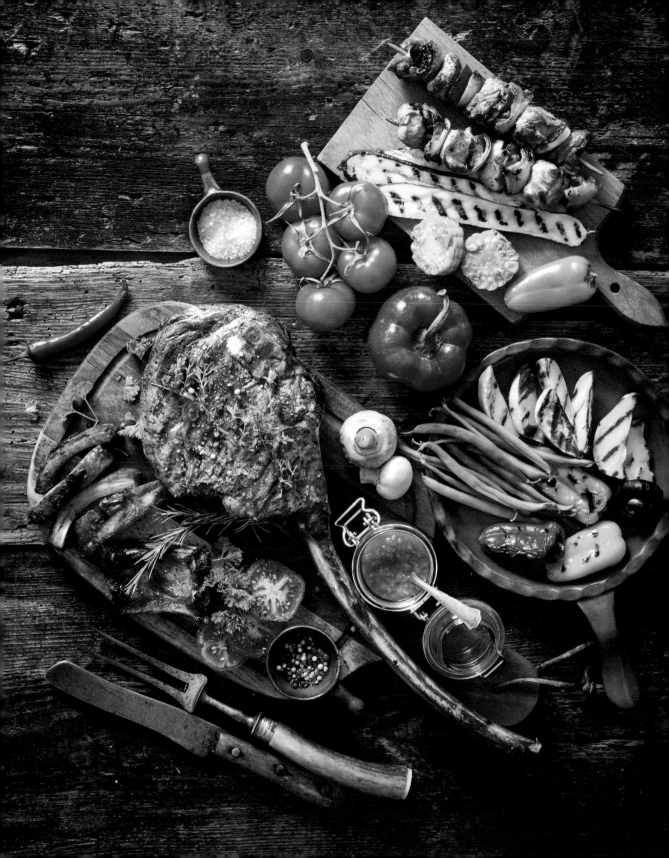

Introduction

You probably picked up this book because you have heard about the widely popular keto diet and how it has helped millions of people lose weight and improve overall health. The documented, short-term benefits of the ketogenic diet include a variety of positive health outcomes in addition to weight loss, including reduced blood sugar, triglycerides, and LDL (bad) cholesterol and increased HDL (good) cholesterol. Animal studies have also suggested that the diet may have antiaging, anti-inflammatory, and cancer-fighting benefits.

We wrote *The 30-Day Keto Plan* to help you achieve your weight-loss and wellness goals safely and efficiently through a user-friendly ketogenic nutrition plan. In addition to offering a selection of unique keto recipes for variation and experimentation, the majority of this book coaches the reader on exactly what to eat for thirty days to produce results as quickly and easily as possible.

The 30-day plan found in this book can be used consecutively, six times in a row, to lose as much as seventy-five pounds within 180 days in a safe manner. Even more important than fewer pounds on the scale, our intention for you is to improve your overall health and wellness via improvements in blood sugar, cholesterol, and triglycerides. Because of this, you will find that we focus our plan on the healthiest anti-inflammatory fats and advise against regular consumption of some common keto-approved foods such as bacon, hot dogs, and pork rinds.

As mentioned in our previous book *Almost Keto*, this healthy fat focus is what I (Aimee) attribute my own well-being to. When I was in my early twenties, my blood test results already revealed that I had high cholesterol. My LDL (bad cholesterol) was far higher than that of my peer group, and I was gaining weight. My father also has bad cholesterol, so the argument that it was genetic made sense. I conceded the fact that I would be on statin drugs by age forty, as predicted by my doctor. With some doubt, I got my blood drawn and cholesterol tested by two other medical professionals while in my twenties and I was given the same verdict—genetically bad cholesterol that could not be changed even if I "became raw vegan." Essentially, I threw in the towel and decided that I would cross that bridge when I got to it, a decade or so later.

It continued to bother me that, by the relatively young age of twenty-nine, I had bad cholesterol and I was gaining weight. This was despite the fact that I had been following most "healthy" mainstream American diet recommendations. I chalked my bad cholesterol luck up to genetics because I ate the way most other people ate. Of course, I determined that this cholesterol problem was something that was out of my control, especially after hearing those words from three different medical professionals.

I relayed my health and weight troubles to my then-boyfriend (and now husband and coauthor) and asked him what his secret was for maintaining a low body fat percentage and perfect blood test results, despite the fact that he is twenty years my senior. His advice, which I found quite counterintuitive at the time? "Eat more fat." This was long before "keto" was a household name, but I took his advice and started modifying my diet, including adding an abundance of healthy fats such as avocado, extra-virgin olive oil, and wild salmon.

Fast-forward to age thirty-eight. I had seen doctors in the preceding decade, but I hadn't specifically gotten tested or asked for results regarding my cholesterol. I was concerned and chose the "out of sight, out of mind" approach. At this point, my son was eighteen months old, and my husband was urging me to get life insurance as a safety net for our family, in case any unforeseen accident or illness should occur. A nurse came to our house to conduct an extensive physical checkup with a full blood panel. I received my results the following month and my husband was the one to open the envelope containing the medical results and the decision from the insurance company. He looked at the results and his first words were, "Your cholesterol!" I turned away, saying "I know, I don't need to hear—" "It's perfect!" he interjected before I could finish. How had this happened, when a decade before, I had been told by medical professionals that the only way I would be able to control my cholesterol in the future would be with drugs?

The most important decision I made to turn my health around was to improve my diet, including adding healthy fats to replace sugar and carbohydrates. The ketogenic diet promotes weight loss from achieving a state of ketosis by consuming a large percentage of fat. It is one of the most popular diets today because it has helped so many people to kick-start their weight loss and transition from the high-sugar, standard American diet to one that includes very little sugar and carbohydrates.

Many people do *not* find the keto diet sustainable for extended periods of time due to the high fat and low carbohydrate intake, and there are still many unanswered questions about the keto diet. There are few studies on the long-term (more than six months) effects of following an extremely high-fat regimen. In addition, several variations of the keto diet exist, some healthier than others. Due to the complexities and unknowns of this fascinating nutrition plan, which dates back to 1923, we highly recommend that this protocol be followed for a short term (no longer than six months) to kick-start your weight-loss goals and obtain freedom from the high-carbohydrate lifestyle.

The 30-Day Keto Plan will reset your nutrition plan and rid you from your cravings for a high-sugar diet. You may achieve your initial desired results in the first thirty days, or you may continue this structured plan for up to six months. Once you have achieved your initial goals, our wean-off plan called Almost Keto (found later in this book) will keep your progress going for years to come, helping you maintain and improve your success in the areas of weight loss and other positive health outcomes, including improved blood sugar and cholesterol levels and a more sustainable and healthier lifestyle.

How to Use this Book as Your 30-Day Guide

There are several nutrition plans found in this book and if you use them all, you will have enough meals and snacks to fill at least sixty days, not just one month! The reason for this is we all like to eat foods in different ways—some of us prefer routine while some of us choose variety. One consistently running theme through all meal plans is simplicity and ease of preparation, while getting the best weight-loss and health results. The last third of this book is dedicated to more creative, in-depth ketogenic recipes which may take more effort in the kitchen. Our goal for you is to complete the first thirty days as easily and effectively as possible, so you can wait to experiment with those recipes if you choose to do so. Or if you want to work in some fancier keto recipes during your first thirty days (like when you have time on the weekends), feel free!

In between the meal plans and recipes, you will find nutrition education information, cited studies, nutrient charts, information about the food industry, lobbying, nutrition myths, and more, so you can learn more about the ketogenic protocol and why it works. As nutritionists, we have had thousands of clients who just want to be instructed on what to eat to get results, because—let's face it—everyone is busy, so finding the time to read an entire book isn't realistic for some. If you fall into this category and just want to know where to look to get your fast and effective meal plans, look here:

- **Chapter (1)** This is where you'll get started with the basics of what you need for your 30-day keto plan. You will be given a very simple meal planning system which introduces you to fast, easy, and relatively inexpensive keto foods that are commonly used— this will be employed to complete the first few days of your plan.

- **Chapter (4)** This is not a meal planning chapter, but, it does detail every food you are allowed to eat during your 30-day keto plan.

- **Chapter (7)** This is where you will be gradually introduced to "batch cooking"—cooking larger portions and storing so you have healthy, ready-to-go meals on hand. You will find three separate three-day meal plans with corresponding grocery lists here.

- **Chapter (8)** This chapter provides what many keto dieters refer to as the "game changer." If you're missing bread, pizza dough, pancakes, and waffles, this chapter gives recipes and meal ideas for these items with keto-approved ingredients.

- **Chapter (10)** Batch cooking in larger amounts will be found in this chapter. You will learn how to make five lunches and dinners for the workweek while choosing an expedited breakfast. Most of the lunch and dinner recipes can be doubled or tripled, and some have the theme of warm saucy casseroles that can easily be refrigerated or frozen and then reheated at a later time.

- **Chapter** (12) This chapter offers a strict intermittent fasting five-day meal plan. This five-day plan tends to offer expedited results, as well as a solution for those who have hit a plateau. You won't find any fancy foods in this chapter, but you'll reap some serious results.

- **Chapter** (14) The "Keto Select" system is found in this chapter and is a "choose your own adventure" style of flexible meal planning that employs the selection of different foods from specific categories to customize your keto-approved meals.

Keep in mind, you may not need to employ all of the above chapters, but since we all have different tastes and preferences, they are there as resources since you may want to customize your meal plan one week, or you may want the convenience of batch cooking for work for the next week. Typically, keto dieters find their preferred way of food preparation and meal planning by trying different tactics, before getting into a simple groove that works for an extended period of time. Congratulations—your new low-sugar lifestyle (and all of the health and weight-loss benefits that come with it) is about to begin!

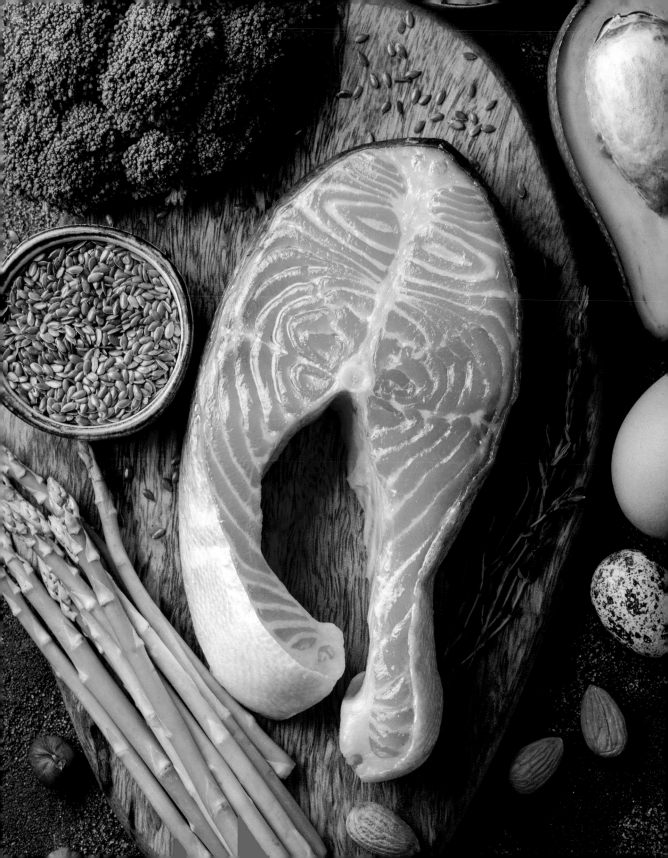

Chapter 1

Let's Get Started—
The First Week of Your
30-Day Keto Plan!

Hello and welcome to your 30-day keto plan! You probably picked up this book because you have some goals in mind, so we don't want to waste any time. Let's dive in and get started. On this first page of this first chapter, we are going to begin the 30-day keto plan process so you can see results as soon as possible. Essentially, the ketogenic (or keto) diet calls for a high fat, low-carbohydrate, moderate-protein food regimen so your body is put in the metabolic state of ketosis, causing it to burn fat for fuel instead of carbohydrates, turning your gut into a fat-burning machine! On average, the keto nutrition plan calls for 70 to 80 percent fat, 5 to 10 percent carbohydrates, and 10 to 20 percent protein for daily caloric intake. For background information and explanations regarding this nutrition plan, you'll find everything you need to know in coming chapters, so feel free to skip ahead if you want to learn more first.

This chapter is your guide to getting started. You'll need to complete three preparation tasks and those are (1) weighing in, (2) taking three "before" photos, and (3) learning the most simple way to keto meal plan. With any process, you need to be able to gauge your results so weighing in to benchmark your starting point is essential. Of course, the number on the scale isn't the only determining factor of progress, so taking a few before pictures, from different angles, will help you see your results in terms of inches and body composition. These tasks will be followed by starting your first few days on the actual 30-day keto program. Your preparation tasks may take one to two days before you start the eating plan, so you will have a little bit of time to get accustomed to the program as you keep reading on about more details, explanations, macronutrient and micronutrient charts, studies, meal plans, grocery lists, and recipes.

Prep Task One: Weighing In

If you don't have a scale, it is beneficial to purchase one so you can track your progress, and it doesn't need to be anything fancy or expensive—just a simple scale that measures your weight. If you have access to a gym scale and you use the gym somewhat regularly, that can work, too. Weight fluctuates throughout the day due to water and food consumption, as well as the clothing we're wearing, so we recommend weighing in first thing in the morning before getting dressed for the day. Jot your weight down or put it in your phone. Consistency is key, so if on your first weigh-in, you stepped on the scale before eating anything and before getting dressed in the morning, be sure to do the same for all further weigh-ins.

Prep Task Two: Taking "Before" Pictures

Sometimes we get just as much (or even more) results from inches lost, opposed to the number on the scale. In addition to weighing in, take three "before" pictures—one frontward facing, one side facing, and one from behind. At the end of the thirty days, you can take the same three pictures so you can visually see the progress you have made. If you want to share your success, hashtag #aimhardnutrition on Instagram and Facebook so everyone can see your results!

Prep Task Three: Learn the Most Simple and Effective Way to Keto Meal Plan

Since you're just beginning your 30-day keto plan, we want to give you a very easy start-up process as the preparation to begin some food plans are so daunting that many put off beginning in the first place! Keep in mind, we have many meal plans, batch-cooking techniques and recipes, meal preparation tactics, and unique keto foods to choose from so days to come will be far more varied, with the option to whip up interesting keto recipes. People are most likely to start a new regimen if it's easy, and that means not dealing with unfamiliar or hard-to-find foods, long preparation times, or expensive kitchen gadgets. We put this simplistic *keto meal planning kit* here in chapter 1, as it is the easiest formula to implement for formatting your keto meals. We urge you to use this kit for at least the first three to five days of your 30-day keto plan to learn the ropes. If you stick to it only for the first seventy-two hours, you will likely still see results on the scale that fast! And if you decide to continue with this meal planning system indefinitely, that is perfectly fine.

Keep It Simple: Keto Meal Planning Kit				
Pick a Protein	Pick a Low-Carb Produce (or two)	Add Two or Three Fats	Pick One Serving of Low-Sugar Fruit Per Day (optional)	Optional Condiments for any Meal
Chicken	Asparagus	Avocado	Blackberries	Fresh or dried herbs and spices
Dairy-based protein (cottage cheese, Greek yogurt, Kefir)	Bell pepper	Avocado oil	Blueberries	Freshly squeezed lemon/lime
Eggs	Broccoli	Avocado oil mayo	Raspberries	Hot sauce
Fish	Broccoli rabe	Bacon	Strawberries	Mustard
Ground beef	Brussels sprouts	Cheese		Sugar-free seasonings
Lamb	Cabbage	Coconut milk		Vinegar
Plant based protein (low-carb, low-sugar)	Cauliflower	Coconut oil		
Pork	Cucumber	Cream		
Shellfish	Eggplant	Eggs		
Steak	Green beans	Grass-fed butter or ghee		
Turkey	Leafy greens/side salad	High-fat, low-carb, low-sugar sauce or dressing		
Venison	Mushrooms	MCT oil		
	Onion (no more than 2 tablespoons per serving, due to carb content)	Nut/seed butters		
	Spaghetti squash	Nuts/seeds		
	Spinach	Olive oil		
	Swiss chard	Olives		
	Tomato	Regular mayo		
	Zucchini	Walnut oil		

For meal examples that employ this chart, you will find five options each for breakfast, lunch, dinner, and snacks below—they are all keto-approved so the guesswork is taken out for you, and you'll be on your way to turn your gut into a fat-burning machine! For the next few days, pick a breakfast, lunch, dinner, and one or two high-fat snacks from the list below, or create your own meals using the chart above.

Breakfast Options

Choose One

2–3 eggs cooked in oil your way, topped with cheese and avocado (both optional) with side of berries or sliced tomatoes.

2–3 egg omelet with sautéed onions, bell pepper, and mushrooms, topped with cheese and avocado (both optional).

2–3 eggs your way with 1–2 pieces of bacon.

Plain Greek yogurt or nondairy yogurt topped with berries and nuts or seeds.

Cottage cheese with berries or tomatoes.

Breakfast box to-go: 1 hard-boiled egg, 1 string cheese, 2–3 ounces smoked salmon, sliced avocado, handful favorite berries.

Lunch Options

Choose One

Green salad topped with chicken or steak, shredded cheese, sliced avocado, olives, oil and vinegar or store-bought ranch or blue cheese dressing (no sugar added).

1–2 cans of tuna or chicken mixed with mayonnaise, mustard, diced celery, and diced red onion. Eat on its own or use celery sticks to dip.

Deli sandwich lettuce wrap: fill one or two large iceberg lettuce cups with your favorite deli meats and cheeses, and any or all of the following: mayonnaise, mustard, avocado, tomato, onion, pickle.

Turkey burger or hamburger with no bun, topped with any or all of the following toppings: cheese, mayonnaise, mustard, avocado, tomato, onion, pickle.

Protein and fat platter: chicken, steak, or fish prepared with any of the following: melted cheese, sliced avocado, sautéed green vegetables, sauerkraut, green salad with oil and vinegar.

Dinner Options

Choose One

Sliced chicken, onion, and bell pepper sautéed in oil and store-bought tomatillo sauce. Top with shredded cheese, sour cream, mashed avocado, and cilantro.

Steak topped with butter, paired with sautéed or roasted asparagus, and small side salad topped with oil and vinegar.

Salmon (or other fish) pan-cooked in grass-fed butter or ghee, paired with steamed cauliflower mashed with Parmesan cheese.

Hamburger (no bun) topped with cheese, mayo, mustard, lettuce, tomato, onion, and avocado paired with green vegetable of choice.

Lamb chops or lamb steak topped with Tzatziki Dipping Sauce (page 265) paired with green vegetable of choice.

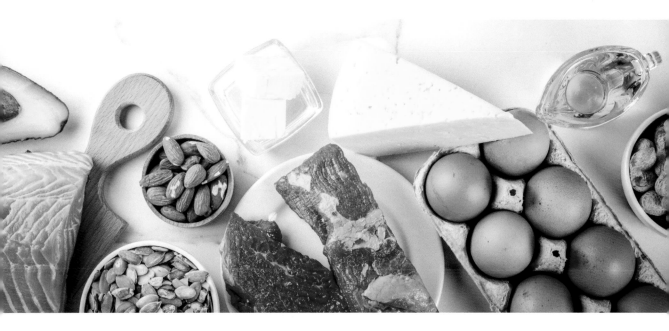

You can repeat meals if you like—for example, if you already have some eggs in the fridge and that means less grocery shopping, have eggs for breakfast on each day. Or if you want to make the tuna/chicken salad ahead of time and have it both days, that's fine too. We want to make the first few days as easy and inexpensive as possible. If this type of simplistic planning works for you (as it does for many!), you can extend this system beyond the first week of your 30-day keto plan. If you want something new and more varied, keep reading on to coming chapters!

High-Fat Snacks
(pick one or two per day)

Serving of nuts or seeds
Piece of cheese
Beef jerky
Celery with nut butter or cream cheese
Hard-boiled egg
2–3 squares dark chocolate (at least 75 percent cacao)
Small Keto Coffee (page 185)
Serving of olives
Half avocado with melted cheese and salsa
Jicama or endive leave with mashed avocado
Sliced cucumber with ranch dressing
Celery with blue cheese dressing
Salami slices with cream cheese and sliced pickles
Coconut cream or half-and-half with raspberries

Portions and Serving Sizes

We do not want you to have to religiously ccount calories and weigh food—essentially, if you stick to the plans in this book, your keto macros will fall into place. Below is a portion guide to help you gauge a sensible portion that is most effective for results. Of course, this is a simplified list of keto foods—if you would like to see everything you can eat, skip forward to chapter 4.

Food	Calories	Visual Cue
Vegetables		
1 cup green vegetables	25	1 baseball
2 cups leafy greens (raw)	25	2 baseballs
Low-Sugar Fruits		
½ cup berries	45	1 tennis ball
½ cup sliced tomato	15	1 tennis ball
½ cup sliced bell pepper	15	1 tennis ball
Fats		
½ cup sliced avocado	115	1 tennis ball
1 tablespoon oil	120	3 dice
1 tablespoon butter	100	3 dice
1 tablespoon ghee	135	3 dice
1 tablespoon mayonnaise	103	3 dice
6 ounces salmon	300	2 decks of cards
1 ounce nuts	160–205	2 golf balls
2 tablespoons nut/seed butter	95–175	1 golf ball
1 cup full-fat yogurt	150	1 baseball
1 cup full-fat cottage cheese	200	1 baseball
1 ounce olives	60	10 whole olives
Proteins		
6 ounces chicken/turkey	200–275	2 decks of cards
6 ounces steak	320	2 decks of cards
6 ounces fish	150–310	2 decks of cards
6 ounces shellfish	130–170	2 hands full
6 ounce ground beef	360	2 decks of cards

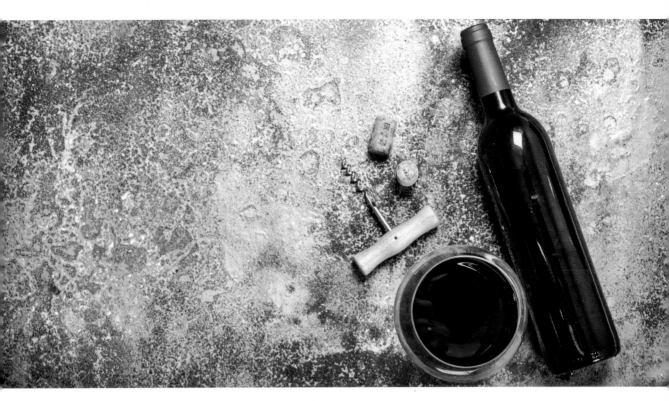

Beverages

As with food, we need to stick to zero-sugar and/or extremely low-sugar beverages during your 30-day plan. Water is always your best bet, however, unsweetened coffee and tea with cream, almond (or other nut) milks, coconut cream, MCT oil, coconut oil, butter, or ghee is keto-approved. Unsweetened sparkling water and bone broth are allowed, as well as 1 to 2 glasses of low-sugar wine (per day) such as cabernet sauvignon, merlot, pinot noir, chardonnay, pinot grigio, and sauvignon blanc with dinner. Rum, whiskey, tequila, vodka, and gin are all keto-friendly, however, they cannot be combined with sugary mixers.

Congratulations on starting your 30-day keto plan! Remember to weigh yourself the morning of your first official day as you will probably see results after the first seventy-two hours. Keep in mind, although the *keto meal planning kit* and basic guidelines found in this chapter are simple, it is the foundation for the ketogenic diet. If you choose to keep using this system for longer than a few days, feel free—it works!

Chapter 2

Why Sugar Addiction Is Common

I f you have taken the big leap and are already on the first week of your 30-day keto plan, congratulations! You have probably noticed that your new way of eating is far lower in sugar and carbohydrates than what you may be used to, and there's a reason for that. Many of us are eating at least three desserts every day, but we don't even realize it. The average American currently consumes fifty-seven pounds of added sugar in one year, which is roughly seventeen teaspoons per day. Compare this sugar intake to an average consumption of two pounds per year, two hundred years ago. Our bodies are simply not built to synthesize the amount of sugar that is commonly used today, resulting in a surge of type 2 diabetes, heart disease, and nonalcoholic fatty liver disease.

You may be thinking it's extreme to state that the average person consumes the equivalent of three desserts per day. While candies, cakes, cookies, and ice cream are obvious examples of sugar culprits, sweeteners are also added to the majority of our packaged foods, fueling the sugar industry's ability to exceed 100 billion dollars in recent years.[1] The industry is so profitable they must defend and downplay the effects of sugar, as illustrated by statements on their own website such as "Sugar is simple, amazingly functional, and it's part of a balanced diet."[2] And yes, sugar can be consumed in true moderation but when you have a 100-billion-dollar industry whose primary interest is profits, our food supply ends up being plagued with a highly unbalanced proportion of sweetened products, making it virtually impossible to escape its presence. It's no surprise our society's health is on the decline when this money-fueled product is the primary culprit

---

1 Dewan, S. "Global Markets for Sugars and Sweeteners in Processed Foods and Beverages." BCC Research, June 2015.

2 "Sugar & The Diet." The Sugar Association. Accessed March 5, 2020. sugar.org/diet/.

for a host of preventable diseases, and since sugar triggers the same responses in the body as some narcotics, it puts us at high risk for long-term addiction.[3]

To give you more clarity about how big this sugar business is, manufacturers add sugar to 74 percent of all of our packaged foods.[4] So even if you tend to skip the traditional dessert foods, you are still (likely) getting far more than the recommended daily intake. An added concern is that our society labels many of these sugar-laden foods as "healthy" which leads the masses down a path of weight gain and sugar-related diseases. How many times have you seen the "heart-healthy" selections on a restaurant menu or the "fit breakfast" at a wellness-based hotel? Let's examine one of these typical meals, which many of us choose in an attempt to start the day off on the right foot.

Heart-Healthy Fit Breakfast Menu

Small plain croissant
Small Fruit, Yogurt, Granola Parfait
Orange Juice

Heart-healthy breakfasts are typically classified by one characteristic and that is being low in fat, meaning less than 3 grams of fat per 100 calories. No other considerations are explored, so we end up with recommended "healthy" fare that has exponential amounts of sugar, and that sugar, if not burned, will turn into fat. Let's break down this breakfast in terms of all macronutrients and sugars.

Food	Calories	Fat (grams)	Carbohydrates (grams)	Protein (grams)	Sugar (grams)
1 croissant	170	6	19	3	5
1 parfait	210	3	40	6	28
1 cup orange juice	110	0	26	2	22
Total	490	9 grams	85 grams	11 grams	55 grams

3 Avena, N., P. Rada, and B. Hoebel. "Evidence for Sugar Addiction: Behavioral and Neurochemical Effects of Intermittent, Excessive Sugar Intake." NCBI. Neuroscience and Biobehavioral Reviews, January 2008. ncbi.nlm.nih.gov/pmc/articles/PMC 2235907/.

4 Ng, S. W., M. M. Slining, & Popkin, B.M. (2012). Use of caloric and noncaloric sweeteners in US consumer packaged foods, 2005–2009. *Journal of the Academy of Nutrition and Dietetics*, 112(11), 1828–1834.e1821-1826.

This one 490-calorie breakfast is packed with 55 grams of sugar, and that far exceeds the daily recommended intake of 37 grams of added sugar per day for men, and 25 for women. The concern is the majority of people would think this is a healthy choice due to the fact that it is low in fat, and devoid of items such as butter and egg yolks. Now add in food and beverages for the remainder of the day and you can easily see how we are consuming several pounds of sugar per year.

When we, as a society, classify unhealthy sugar-laden meals like this as a good choice, it's no wonder people are confused about what to eat for weight loss and optimal wellness. Seventy-four percent of our packaged foods have added sugars, and, since the Food and Drug Administration does not regulate terms such as "natural," "superfood," or "premium," we may falsely perceive many of these processed foods as conducive to weight loss and health. Several variations of the following supposed health food items tend to have the highest amounts of sugars despite the fact they are usually touted as being healthy, so it is important to always check the label for nutrition information, ingredients, and sugar content.

Flavored Yogurts

Some yogurts can be incorporated into your ketogenic plan, but you must have a good look at the nutrition and ingredients label to ensure you're not packing in the same amount of sugar (or sometimes more) as you would with a bowl of ice cream. Flavored and low- or nonfat yogurts tend to be the biggest offenders with upward of 47 grams of sugar per cup, which exceeds the limit of daily sugar intake for men and women in just one serving. It is best to choose full-fat, plain yogurt and be sure to check the label to make sure there is no added sugar by way of high-fructose corn syrup or other sweeteners.

Protein Bars

Just like yogurt, some protein bars are formulated to meet ketogenic standards, but the majority are not. Many contain as much as 30 grams of sugar per bar which is equivalent to eating a standard candy bar. If you do enjoy snacking on a protein bar, check the label for high fat content and extremely low sugar content—typically, these keto-friendly protein bar ingredients include items such as coconut oil, almond butter, cocoa butter, medium-chain triglyceride (MCT) oil, and collagen.

Granola
Granola tends to be classified as a nutritious health food but most commercial brands include a variety of sweeteners in one brand. All three—cane sugar, brown rice syrup, and tapioca syrup—are found in popular commercial brands of granola. Unfortunately, it is common to top flavored yogurt with these sweetened grain mixtures, resulting in a small meal that contains as much as 63 grams of sugar. If you're a granola fan, there are many keto renditions that include ingredients such as nuts, seeds, coconut, coconut oil, and vanilla extract.

Kombucha
Kombucha is ancient fermented tea and provides a host of benefits through its probiotic content, however, some brands have as much as 20 grams of sugar per serving, which is almost comparable to the sugar content of soda. If you're looking for the gut and microbiome benefits that kombucha can provide, choose unflavored selections that have less than 4 grams of sugar per serving.

Cereal Bars
Like cereal, cereal bars are touted as "heart healthy" yet are packed with added sugars and highly processed ingredients. The nutritional value of the processed ingredients is so low that most cereal bars are fortified with fake synthetic nutrients as the processing kills many of the naturally occurring vitamins and minerals.

Premade Soups
Soups are a wonderful part of the keto nutrition plan when using ingredients such as coconut milk, avocado, vegetables, and proteins, however, if you're looking for a quick low-carbohydrate and low-sugar soup found in a can, you will really have to inspect the nutrition label. For example, one can of Campbell's classic tomato soup has 20 grams of

sugar—the same as two glazed donuts! Not all canned soups are sugar culprits, so with some label checking, you may be able to find some convenient options.

Vitamin Water

Vitamin water is marketed as healthy since it contains a variety of added synthetic nutrients (some of which can be hard to absorb). Another addition to these drinks is sugar—one bottle has as much as 32 grams, which is comparable to the amount of sugar found in soda. It's best to stick to water or unsweetened sparkling water during your 30-day keto plan.

Canned Baked Beans

Beans and legumes aren't regularly consumed in the keto world, however, if you're on point with measuring your carbohydrate intake, you may be able to squeeze a small portion in. This doesn't mean canned baked beans, though! Canned baked beans are known for their sweet and tangy flavor because only ½ cup packs 10 grams of sugar. Opt for dried beans that you have to prepare yourself so you know there are no added ingredients.

Bottled Smoothies

Many brands of bottled smoothies have more sugar than soda, and the misleading factor is their labels are allowed to say "no added sugars." This is because the sugar technically comes from fruit. However, when several pieces of fruit are processed, stripping their nutrients, and condensed into a bottle, your body cannot decipher this type of sugar from the type found in a candy bar. Smoothies are a part of the keto nutrition plan, but opt for ingredients such as coconut milk, kefir, avocado, hemp seeds, kale, and berries.

Our society's classification of what is healthy, in addition to actual health foods that have now succumbed to the sugar industry by being altered into sweeter variations, are two driving factors that are contributing to our sugar addictions. Another concern is that our own government's guidelines are contributing to this sugar pandemic as well. The USDA MyPlate has made some small improvements when compared to 1992's famous (and faulty)

Food Pyramid, which suggested eating six to eleven servings of high-glycemic grains per day, as well as very little fat, despite how beneficial healthy fats are. However, many of the dietary guidelines for Americans still reek of monetary interests as opposed to the interests of the health of our public. To the right is an example day of food that meets the USDA MyPlate's dietary recommendations for a 2,000-calorie diet.

One may look at these recommendations and nod at the fact that they seem "normal" for today's standards and, yes, they are normal; however, they are extremely faulty and actually contribute to serious medical conditions that run rampant in today's population, such as excessive weight gain and type 2 diabetes. Let's take this recommended daily intake of food and break it down into macronutrients (carbohydrates, protein, fat), as well as sugar so we can get a better understanding of the implications of these suggested foods.

USDA MyPlate Daily Recommended Foods and Servings (2,000-calorie diet)

3 cups of nonfat or low-fat milk
2 pieces of bread
1 cup of cereal
1 cup of pasta
1 cup of orange juice
1 cup of sliced bananas
1 cup of sweet potatoes
1 cup of broccoli
½ cup of carrots
4 ounces of chicken
1 egg
1 tablespoon of peanut butter

Food	Carbohydrates (grams)	Protein (grams)	Fat (grams)	Sugar (grams)
Whole wheat bread (2 slices)	24	8	2	4
Whole-grain cereal (1 cup)	29	3	2	7
Whole wheat pasta (1 cup)	41	7	2	2
Baked sweet potato (1 cup)	41	4	0	13
Broccoli (1 cup)	9	3	0	2
Carrots (½ cup)	6	0	2	2
Sliced banana (1 cup)	34	2	0	18
Orange juice (1 cup)	26	2	0	22
Chicken (4 ounces)	0	30	4	0
1 egg	1	6	5	0
1 tablespoon peanut butter	3	4	8	2
2% milk (3 cups)	36	24	15	36
Totals	**250 grams**	**93 grams**	**40 grams**	**108 grams**

As you can see, this suggested example of one day of "healthy food" results in 108 grams of sugar, as well as an abundance of high-glycemic carbohydrates, many of which come from processed foods. To put it into perspective, this amount of sugar and carbohydrates is equivalent to eating almost eleven glazed donuts in one day! One may say that sugars from the above-listed foods are different than refined sugar; unfortunately, your body is negatively affected by too much sugar, whether it is from a natural source or from a donut. Another possible argument is that these foods do offer a variety of nutritional benefits (unlike eleven glazed donuts), thus justifying the sugar and carbohydrate intake. We will explain in later chapters how to get twice the nutrients offered by this typical plan, while consuming a fraction of the sugar, and no high-glycemic, processed carbohydrates (your carbs will come from healthier sources)!

The 108 grams of sugar found in the above government-recommended plan leads to the next contributing factor of our sugar addictions. The USDA MyPlate sample meal plan is considered healthy despite having 108 grams of sugar because the "added sugars" do not exceed 10 percent of the daily caloric intake. Added sugars include sugars that are added during the processing of foods, such as white sugar, brown sugar, corn sweetener, corn syrup, dextrose, fructose, glucose, high-fructose corn syrup, honey, lactose, malt syrup, maltose, molasses, raw sugar, and sucrose. These added sugars do not include naturally occurring sugars from items such as fruits (fructose) and milk (lactose). What's not being taken into consideration is the fact that the cumulative effect of regular consumption of fructose and lactose, as well as carbohydrates from foods such as breads, cereals, pastas, and potatoes, do have adverse effects on blood sugar and maintaining ideal weight.

In 2016, the FDA amended the requirements for the nutrition label, mandating the listed amounts of added sugars. On one hand, this is a wonderful tool to visualize exactly how much sugar has been added to things like cookies, ice cream, sauces, dressings, and beverages, however, it can also create a false sense of health for a variety of other problematic food choices. If one were faced with a 16-ounce orange soda drink with a label exhibiting 58 grams of added sugar versus a 16-ounce orange juice with a label exhibiting 0 added sugars (while still including 48 grams of natural sugar), the "healthy" choice would be the orange juice, as that sugar is "natural." To take this a step further, one may now choose a fruit smoothie, which typically has even more sugar than soda, but just as the orange juice, the label will exhibit no added sugars.

Unfortunately, the FDA's added sugar label leaves out key information that is detrimental to our health. It does not recognize the fact that the sugars from initial natural fruit sources have been heavily concentrated and processed during production. During this processing, the fruit's properties have been significantly altered, notably the stripping of fiber and concentration of juice from several pieces of fruit into one small bottle. This process greatly affects the way our bodies process the sugar which has key implications for our health, all while leading the consumer to believe he or she is making a healthy choice.[5]

We also come across this same "added sugars" versus "natural sugars" confusion on the nutrition label of dairy products. Lactose, the natural sugar found in milk has conflicting research regarding how it affects our blood sugar levels. Lactose can, in fact, raise blood glucose levels, however, some nutritionists argue that lactose converts to blood glucose relatively slowly due to the fact that the enzyme lactase slowly splits up glucose into galactose, leading to a slower glycemic response. Other nutrition and medical professionals say that even though dairy has a lower glyemic index ranking, it still stimulates insulin as if it had a high glycemic index ranking. This is due to the combination of milk's amino acids found in whey proteins with the lactose. This combination leads some doctors to say that milk's insulin response is actually extreme and should be avoided if one is looking for optimal blood sugar levels.[6]

We have discussed three highly concerning issues that greatly contribute to Americans' collective sugar addiction, as they are very convoluted due to their ambiguous

---

5   Marty Micsmeanderings, Evan Lavizadeh, Alireza, Bryan A. Matsumoto, Emily Marco, et al. "Natural and Added Sugars: Two Sides of the Same Coin," October 5, 2015. sitn.hms.harvard.edu/flash/2015/natural-and-added-sugars-two-sides-of-the-same-coin/.

6   Spero, David. "Is Milk Bad for You? Diabetes and Milk." Management. Diabetes Self Management, June 20, 2017. diabetes-selfmanagement.com/blog/is-milk-bad-for-you-diabetes-and-milk/.

nature. These three findings have a huge impact on the vast majority of the population due to the abundance of use of these hidden-sugar characteristics.

- Manufacturers add sugar to 74 percent of our packaged foods.
- Society labels many sugar-laden foods and nutrition plans as "healthy."
- Natural sugars found in processed foods are looked at as safely consumed as they do not fall in the "added sugar" category, despite having the same health implications as added sugars.

The one and only definitive sugar guideline we are given by the Food and Drug Administration is to limit added sugar intake to 50 grams or less per day, based on a 2,000-calorie diet. Ironically, there is no daily recommended intake for total sugars (added sugars plus natural sugars) because no agency has made the specific recommendation for the amount of total sugars to eat in one day. So essentially, if one consumes 29 grams of added sugars from an 8-ounce soda, 9 grams of added sugar in a serving of Honey Nut Cheerios, 8 grams of added sugar in two tablespoons of barbecue sauce, and 4 grams of added sugar in salad dressing, he has remained within the limit of what is deemed a healthy sugar intake by the FDA. Simply adding two sources of natural sugars—milk with the cereal and a fruit smoothie later in the day—brings our total sugars to roughly 120 grams. At the beginning of this chapter, we gave the statistic of 57 pounds of added sugar consumed per year by the average American, but we didn't say how many pounds of total sugars (added plus natural) consumed on average because that number isn't gauged or monitored since we are not given a guideline for total sugar intake. As nutritionists, we have worked with thousands of clients and have compiled their daily food log questionnaires to try to get a better idea of average total sugar intake—to the right is an example of a meal plan that incorporates the most common meals and snacks.

Standard American Diet Meal Plan

Breakfast
Coffee with flavored creamer
Raisin Bran cereal with milk
1 medium banana

Lunch
Turkey sandwich
Chips
Snapple flavored iced tea

Dinner
Chicken with side of pasta and vegetables

Dessert
Serving of ice cream

Food	Carbohydrates (grams)	Protein (grams)	Fat (grams)	Sugar (grams)
Coffee with flavored creamer (2 tablespoons)	10	0	3	10
Raisin Bran cereal (1 cup)	46	5	2	18
2% milk (1 cup)	12	8	5	12
1 medium banana	23	1	0	12
Whole wheat bread (2 pieces)	24	8	2	4
Turkey deli meat (2 pieces)	2	7	1	1
Cheese (1 piece)	1	5	9	1
Lettuce, tomato, onion, mustard	6	0	0	2
Chips (1 small bag)	15	2	10	0
Snapple peach-flavored iced tea (16-ounce bottle)	40	0	0	40
Chicken (5 ounces)	0	30	4	0
Broccoli (1 cup)	9	3	0	2
Whole wheat pasta (1 cup)	41	7	2	2
Chocolate ice cream (⅔ cup)	23	3	11	22
Totals	**252 grams**	**79 grams**	**49 grams**	**126 grams**

This common meal plan that, as you can see, isn't overly extreme with an abundance of sodas, desserts, fried foods, and fast foods, is still not conducive for weight management or health with 126 grams of sugar (or 30 teaspoons). While some of the sugar content comes from natural sources, this combination of added sugars and natural sugars still results in an overload that is not meant to be tolerated in our bodies. You can assume this sugar number is twofold if one drinks soda regularly and/or indulges in office donuts and cookies, or makes an afternoon run to the local coffee shop with a calorie-ridden pick-me-up.

We want this 30-day plan to help you combat our oversweetened food supply. If you have a sugar addiction, you're not alone as overcoming the obstacles that have been put in front of us is quite daunting since we can't seem to get away from it—sugar is, in fact, everywhere. On that note, one thing you will find a little different about this book is that we do not have any fancy dessert recipes for you. You won't find a list of keto-friendly sweeteners, either. We want you to kick your sugar habit and the need for sweet foods to be content. You can make it through these thirty days and when you do, you'll realize how much sugar was in your diet before and you won't want to return.

Chapter 3

The Ketogenic Diet, Explained

The *30-Day Keto Plan* is meant as a restart to put perspective on how much sugar we may truly be consuming on a regular basis. Most people who succeed with getting through a strict low-sugar regimen for just one month end up creating better, long-lasting nutrition habits. We don't intend for you to stick to this regimen for extended periods of time (although some choose to do so) and we do have a wean-off plan for you, found later in this book. Essentially, we need to rewire our brains with regard to the way we think about and use food, and reverse the high-sugar habits that have been instilled in us all by the food industry for the past several decades.

You may be wondering, *why are we told, by trusted governmental sources, to eat these foods if they may lead us down a path of type 2 diabetes, weight gain, and heart disease?* The United States Department of Agriculture plays a heavy role in determining these recommendations and then these same guidelines are incorporated in the nutrition education curriculum that is taught to nutritionists, as well as some doctors. Essentially, as opposed to being based on scientific research and evidence, these recommendations are influenced by food producers, manufacturers, and special interest groups. One of the USDA's largest priorities is to strengthen and support the food, agriculture, and farming industries so these guidelines may be disproportionately based on profit as opposed to the health of the general population.[1]

Every year, the food industry donates millions of dollars to politicians who are in charge of making decisions regarding food regulation. This results in the industry's ability to market foods that are laden with sugar, salt, calories, and unhealthy fats. For

---

1   Nestle, M. "Food Lobbies, the Food Pyramid, and U.S. Nutrition Policy." NCBI. July 1, 1993. Accessed February 16, 2019. ncbi .nlm.nih.gov/pubmed/8375951.

example, the United States Department of Health and Human Services, as well as the USDA, vetoed their own expert panel's suggestions to reduce processed meat and sugary beverage consumption in their 2015–2020 Dietary Guidelines, despite substantial evidence that those items are harmful to public health.[2] Through this orchestration of campaign funding and lobbying, the food industry has effectively quashed and avoided evidence-based guidelines and taxation. Therefore, the industry has been somewhat allowed to market, formulate, and sell foods that are proven to be detrimental to health when consumed in excess.

In addition to our own regulatory agencies, who should be protecting our health by providing accurate information regarding nutrition, we have product powerhouses such as Coca-Cola that have donated millions of dollars to researchers whose intentions are to downplay the effects of sugary beverages on weight gain. Of course, we may expect this sort of underhanded activity when it comes to a large corporation that is trying to market its products, but we don't necessarily expect it from Harvard scientists. Back in the 1960s, Harvard scientists were paid by the sugar industry to minimize the link between heart disease and sugar. They had to name a new supposed culprit to take sugar's place, and that scapegoat was fat.[3] Unfortunately this faulty, money-based science has been the foundation for a variety of nutrition guidelines throughout the past five decades and has led the masses down a path of falsehoods when considering sugar, carbohydrate, and fat intake in their daily nutrition regimens.

The high-fat, low-sugar ketogenic diet has actually been around for almost 200 years. In the nineteenth century, the ketogenic diet was used to treat diabetes, and it began to be used in the 1920s to treat drug-resistant epilepsy in children. Not just an effective weight-loss trend, keto is still being used in that treatment capacity, and is also being investigated as a potential breakthrough treatment for an array of neurological disorders

---

2   Gostin, Lawrence O. ""Big Food" Is Making America Sick." NCBI. September 13, 2013. Accessed March 7, 2019. ncbi.nlm.nih.gov /pmc/articles/PMC5020160/

3   Damle, S. G. "Smart Sugar? The Sugar Conspiracy." NCBI. July 24, 2017. Accessed March 7, 2019. ncbi.nlm.nih.gov/pmc/articles /PMC5551319/.

and disease. The general idea of the keto diet is to remain extremely low in carbohydrates while consuming an extremely high percentage of fat, so your body can be put into a metabolic state of ketosis. This state of ketosis causes the liver to produce ketones, resulting in your body becoming efficient in burning fat (instead of carbohydrates) for energy.

There is no single standard ketogenic diet with a concrete ratio of macronutrients (carbohydrates, protein, fat), as the required levels of macronutrients for ketosis can vary from person to person.[4] Typically speaking, the keto nutrition plan calls for a total carbohydrate intake of less than 50 grams per day, and it can be as low as 20 grams per day. Popular ketogenic resources suggest an average of 70 to 80 percent fat from total daily calories, 5 to 10 percent carbohydrates, and 10 to 20 percent protein. Within these ranges, for a 2,000-calorie diet, this calculates to around 155 to 177 grams of fat, 25 to 50 grams of total carbohydrates, and 50 to 100 grams of protein.

To take the guesswork out, on the next page is a table that shows how many grams of fat, protein, and carbohydrates you need from a variety of daily caloric intake requirements, starting with 1,200 per day and ending with 3,000 per day. Although the mainstream average number of calories to consume is 2,000 a day, that number is wrong for many people, as required calories are determined by current weight, goal weight, gender, age, and activity level. Free calorie calculators can be accessed online so you can determine what is best for you and your goals.

---

4 "Diet Review: Ketogenic Diet for Weight Loss." The Nutrition Source, May 22, 2019. hsph.harvard.edu/nutrition source/healthy -weight/diet-reviews/ketogenic-diet/.

Total Calories	Fat Calories	Grams of Fat	Protein Calories	Grams of Protein	Carbohydrate Calories	Grams of Carbohydrates	Daily Total
1,200	840–960	93–107	120–240	30–60	60–120	15–30	1,200 Calories 93–107 grams fat 30–60 grams protein 15–30 grams carbs
1,500	1,050–1,200	117–133	150–300	38–75	75–150	19–38	1,500 Calories 116–133 grams fat 38–75 grams protein 19–38 grams carbs
2,000	1,400–1,600	156–178	200–400	50–100	100–200	25–50	2,000 Calories 156–178 grams fat 50–100 grams protein 25–50grams carbs
2,500	1,750–2,000	194–222	250–500	63–125	125–250	31–63	2,500 Calories 194–222 grams fat 63–125 grams protein 31–63 grams carbs
3,000	2,100–2,400	233–267	300–600	75–150	150–300	38–75	3,000 Calories 233–267 grams fat 75–100 grams protein 38–75 grams carbs

Net Carbohydrates Versus Total Carbohydrates

You will hear talk of "net carbohydrate" in the ketogenic world. Total carbohydrate limits found in the table above account for straight-up carbohydrate totals as listed on the nutrition label. Net carbohydrates are found by subtracting the grams of fiber (which are indigestible carbohydrates) from the grams of carbohydrates. For example, a serving of cauliflower contains 5 grams of carbohydrates and 2 grams of fiber, so you simply subtract 2 from 5 and that gives you 3 grams of net carbohydrates. Some circles in the keto community also advise to subtract grams of sugar alcohols (in addition to the grams of fiber) from the grams of carbohydrates to get net carbohydrates. Other circles advise against this, as many studies show that sugar alcohols actually do get absorbed into the bloodstream to some extent, affecting blood glucose levels. As we have mentioned before, this book is all about kicking the sugar habit, so none of our recipes incorporate sugar alcohols, so you can simply subtract grams of fiber from grams of carbohydrates to get your net carbohydrate count. If you count total carbohydrates as per the nutrition label, you can follow the table above. If you choose to take the "net carbohydrate" route, an average rule of thumb to follow is to not exceed 25 grams of net carbohydrates per day.

To achieve this breakdown of macronutrients in the standard ketogenic diet, there tend to be two different ways keto dieters approach their nutrition plans. Some adhere to the healthiest keto foods, while others choose unhealthier keto foods such as bacon, hot dogs, pork rinds, and low-carbohydrate fast food meals. And of course, some people may do a combination of both. We strongly advise to stick to the healthiest keto foods (found in chapter 4) as closely as possible, while only allowing a little bit of leeway for unhealthier fare, as weight loss is not the only intention—overall health is just as important (if not more)! On the next page you will find a sample ketogenic meal plan that follows these healthy guidelines:

- Whole foods with minimal processing
- No fast food
- Limited deli/processed meats
- Quality oils
- Majority of carbohydrates from green vegetables
- Extremely low-sugar fruits
- Healthy fats from avocado, nuts, salmon, egg yolks, and oils
- Quality proteins from organic, wild, and grass-fed sources if available
- At least 25 grams of fiber per day
- No more than 1,500 milligrams of sodium per day.

Sample One-Day Meal Plan

Breakfast: Two whole eggs scrambled (using extra-virgin olive oil) and side of raspberries. Coffee with cream.

Snack: Macadamia nuts.

Lunch: Bunless cheeseburger topped with avocado, lettuce, tomato, onion, and mustard.

Snack: Celery with almond butter.

Dinner: Salmon with coconut oil-sautéed spinach and broccoli.

Food	Calories	Fat (grams)	Protein (grams)	Net Carbs (grams)	Sodium (milligrams)	Fiber (grams)	Sugar (grams)
Eggs (2 whole)	156	10	12	1	124	0	0
Extra-virgin olive oil (1 tbsp.)	119	14	0	0	0	0	0
Raspberries (½ cup)	33	0	0	3	0	4	2.5
Macadamia nuts (¼ cup)	240	25	3	2	2	3	0
70% lean ground beef (5 oz.)	465	40	20	0	95	0	0
Cheddar cheese (1 slice)	113	9	7	0	174	0	0
½ avocado	161	15	2	2	7	7	0.5
Lettuce, tomato, onion, mustard	25	0	1	3	120	2	1
Celery (2 stalks)	11	0	1	1	64	1	0
Almond butter (2 tbsp.)	196	18	7	3	2	3	1
Salmon (6 oz.)	300	18	28	0	85	0	0
Cooked spinach (½ cup)	23	0	3	1.5	0	2.5	0
Coconut oil (1 tbsp.)	117	14	0	0	0	0	0
Broccoli (1 cup)	62	0	3	7	60	5	1.5
Totals	2,021 calories	163 grams	87 grams	24 grams	733 milligrams	28 grams	7 grams

The basis of the keto diet in terms of weight loss is that if you do not feed the body glucose (sugar) obtained through carbohydrates, which is the primary source of energy for the body's cells, an alternative fuel is produced from stored fat, and that fuel is referred to as "ketones." When very small amounts of carbohydrates are consumed, the body first takes stored glucose from the liver and only temporarily breaks down muscles. If this process continues for three to five days and the stored glucose gets completely depleted, insulin levels decrease, and the body starts to use fat as fuel. This results in the liver producing ketone bodies from fat, which can be used for energy in place of glucose.[5] Numerous studies have shown the keto diet to assist with weight loss and blood sugar level improvements, however, the exact reasons as to why the keto diet can produce weight loss and blood sugar improvement is still up for debate.[6] Some research-based theories are as follows:

- Food cravings are lowered due to the satiety of consuming high-fat foods.
- Appetite-stimulating hormones such as insulin and ghrelin are decreased when low amounts of carbohydrates are consumed.
- Ketone bodies (which are the main source of fuel) reduce the feeling of hunger.
- Increased calorie burning resulting from metabolic effects of obtaining glucose from fat and protein conversion.
- Decreased insulin levels resulting in promotion of fat loss, as opposed to lean body mass loss.

5   "Diet Review: Ketogenic Diet for Weight Loss." The Nutrition Source, May 22, 2019. hsph.harvard.edu/nutritionsource/healthy-weight/diet-reviews/ketogenic-diet/.

6   Paoli, Antonio. "Ketogenic Diet for Obesity: Friend or Foe?" NCBI. February 01, 2014. Accessed March 23, 2019. ncbi.nlm.nih.gov/pmc/articles/PMC3945587/.

How to Measure Ketones in the Body

Some keto dieters want to track the state of progress by measuring the amounts of ketones the liver is producing to ensure the metabolic state of ketosis is being achieved. This is certainly not required, but if you're curious how to do it, the following options are available. The three primary ways to measure ketones are via the blood, breath, and urine, and they are detailed below.

Blood glucose test: A simple blood test through the prick of a finger is the most accurate way to measure ketones. Be sure to wash your hands or disinfect with alcohol before the test, and it is helpful to prick the side of the finger, where it's less sensitive. The ideal range to look for is between 0.5 and 5mM/L.

Breath analyzer: Breath analyzers do not tell you your exact ketone level, however, they do provide a range to determine whether or not you are in ketosis. Some argue this form of testing is more reliable than the use of urine strips, however, it is not 100 percent accurate.

Urine strips: Testing the urine measures the presence of acetoacetate (the first ketone produced in the body during ketosis). The darker the color of the test strip, the more ketones are present. This test can have false positives and negatives, so some in the keto community don't recommend this method as a preferred choice, but it does work for many.

Other Possibilities for Keto Weight Loss That Are Not Necessarily Attributed to Ketone Levels

Let's say you don't measure your ketones—you most certainly can get amazing results as the ketogenic diet is extremely low in sugar and carbohydrates and that is key since sugar and carbohydrates turn to fat, if not burned. The four following strategies, which are, coincidentally, characterized by the 30-day keto plan, will contribute to substantial health and weight loss efforts.

Consuming Less Sugar

Sugar consumption is the primary culprit of weight gain, type 2 diabetes, and a host of other ailments. The average American consumes 71 grams (or 17 teaspoons) of added sugar per day, which translates into 57 pounds of added sugar per year, per person. When one shifts from the standard high-sugar American diet to one that is very low in sugar, weight loss and blood sugar improvements will naturally follow.

Consuming Fewer Carbohydrates

Like with sugar, when one adopts a dietary regimen that is substantially lower in carbohydrates, results will follow. The average person consumes 260 grams of carbohydrates per day, so when that number is cut exponentially, less sugar will be consumed as carbohydrates convert into sugar, and sugar turns into fat if not burned.

Consuming Fewer Calories

Consuming less sugar and carbohydrates will, of course, lead to lower calorie consumption. When we eliminate or limit "filler" foods such as sugary beverages with a meal, dessert following dinner, and empty-calorie main courses and side dishes, we will naturally consume fewer calories, and these calories will be more nutrient-dense, providing the fuel we need for a healthy lifestyle.

Eating Consciously

When a new dietary regimen is employed, we consciously choose to eat foods that are beneficial for weight loss and overall well-being, instead of maintaining the status quo of the standard American diet and eating what we always ate before.

The four above-mentioned characteristics that are proven weight-loss tactics happen to be the same traits found in *The 30-Day Keto Plan*. The majority of people who go from the standard American diet of hundreds of grams of carbohydrates per day should definitely see results soon after changing to the ketogenic protocol. The following chapter outlines everything you can eat during your 30-day keto plan, and you'll be pleasantly surprised by the variety!

Chapter 4

Everything You Can Eat

This chapter is your go-to guide for everything you can and can't eat for the next thirty days. The meal plans found in coming chapters do not include every single item in the following "can" list, however, more options are listed in case you are looking for a variety of additions. We urge you to eat the healthiest keto-approved foods to achieve overall well-being in addition to your weight-loss goals.

Vegetables

If you're unsure of which vegetables are best when making a grocery run, sticking to selections that are green is a rule to keep in mind. If you don't see your favorite(s) on the list, you can add them if green in color. Otherwise, check to see if each serving has 5 grams or less of net carbohydrates.

Fruits

Some low-sugar fruits are allowed on the ketogenic plan, and some are so low in sugar that many think they're vegetables. Many fruits such as pineapple, mango, and grapes contain high amounts of fructose, which affects our bodies in a similar manner as table sugar, so it is imperative to eliminate high-glycemic fruits while adhering to the keto plan.

A Note About Organic Produce

There is a handful of keto-approved vegetables and fruits that fall into the "dirty dozen" category, meaning they have the highest levels of pesticides. If possible, it is best to purchase the organic variations of these "dirty dozen" selections, and we have highlighted those for you.

A Note About Onions

A 100-gram (⅔ cup) serving of onions/shallots can have as much as 17 grams of carbohydrates, but the manner in which we typically eat onions calls for much less than 100 grams. When sprinkling onions on a salad or sautéing shallots for a sauce, the carbohydrate count is still low enough to be keto-approved. If you're eating a roasted vegetable mixture, try not to exceed more than ½ cup of onions.

Vegetables

- Artichokes
- Arugula
- Asparagus
- Bok choy
- Broccoli
- Broccoli rabe
- Brussels sprouts
- Cabbage/sauerkraut
- Cauliflower
- Celery
- Chard
- Chicory greens
- Endive
- Fennel bulb
- Green beans
- Hot peppers
- Kale
- Kohlrabi
- Lettuces
- Mushrooms
- Onions
- Radishes
- Seaweed
- Spinach
- Swiss chard
- Watercress

Fruits

- Avocados
- Bell peppers (any color)
- Blackberries
- Blueberries
- Cucumbers/pickles
- Eggplant
- Lemons
- Limes
- Olives
- Pumpkin
- Raspberries
- Spaghetti squash
- Strawberries
- Tomatoes
- Zucchini

A Note About Berries

Berries are the higher-sugar and higher-carbohydrate selections of keto-approved fruits, however, they are packed with essential micronutrients, fiber, and antioxidants, so they are a healthy addition to anyone's diet. Since we are trying to remain extremely low in sugar and carbohydrates, this table will help you be mindful of your berry intake.

50-gram (½ cup) serving		
Berry Type	**Total Carbs**	**Net Carbs**
Blackberries	5 grams	2.5 grams
Raspberries	6 grams	2.5 grams
Strawberries	4 grams	3 grams
Blueberries	10.5 grams	8.5 grams

Proteins

You will find a variety of keto-friendly animal proteins in this section and some selections can also double as fats as they are high in both protein and fat macronutrients. All animal proteins that have a substantial fat content are marked as such for your convenience.

Dairy

Most dairy components have adequate amounts of fat, while remaining very low in carbohydrates. While you can incorporate cottage cheese, Greek yogurt, and kefir in moderation, they are highlighted in orange as they are higher in carbohydrates than other dairy selections.

Nuts, Seeds, Nut Butters, Seed Butters

Some nuts and seeds are lower in carbohydrates and higher in fat, making them better keto choices, however, all selections here are allowed on the keto nutrition plan. The highest fat and lowest carbohydrate selections are Brazil nuts, macadamia nuts, pecans, and walnuts (highlighted in the following list), while the highest in carbohydrates are cashews and pistachios. All others fall somewhere in between.

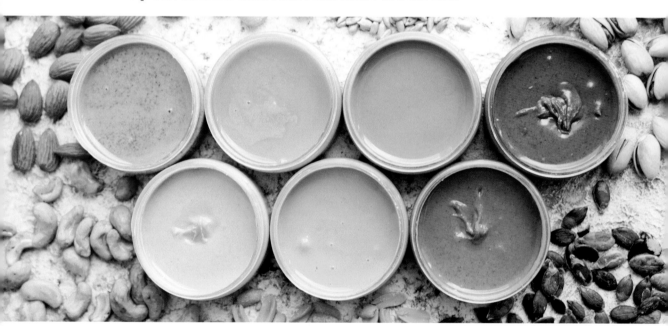

Poultry

- Chicken
- Chicken with skin
- Duck
- Game hen
- Pheasant
- Quail
- Rabbit
- Turkey
- Turkey with skin

Eggs

- Chicken eggs
- Duck eggs
- Goose eggs
- Quail eggs

Red Meat

- Beef
- Boar
- Buffalo
- Elk
- Goat
- Lamb
- Pork/Bacon/ Sausage
- Venison

Seafood

- Anchovies
- Bass
- Carp
- Catfish
- Clams
- Cod
- Crab
- Flounder
- Haddock
- Halibut
- Herring
- Lobster
- Mackerel
- Mussels
- Octopus
- Oysters
- Prawns
- Salmon
- Sardines
- Scallops
- Snails
- Snapper
- Sole
- Swordfish
- Trout
- Tuna
- Walleye

Dairy

- Butter and ghee (clarified butter)
- Cheeses
  Blue cheese
  Brie
  Camembert
  Cheddar
  Cottage cheese (full-fat)
  Cream cheese (full-fat)
  Feta
  Goat cheese
  Gouda
  Gruyère
  Mascarpone
  Mozzarella
  Muenster
  Parmesan
  Provolone
  Ricotta
  Swiss
- Greek yogurt (full-fat)
- Half-and-half
- Heavy whipping cream
- Kefir
- Sour cream (full-fat)

Nuts and Seeds

- Almonds
- Brazil nuts
- Cashews
- Coconut (unsweetened)
- Hazelnuts
- Macadamia nuts
- Peanuts
- Pecans
- Pili nuts
- Pine nuts
- Pistachios
- Walnuts
- Chia seeds
- Flax seeds
- Hemp seeds
- Poppy seeds
- Pumpkin seeds
- Sesame seeds
- Sunflower seeds
- Almond butter
- Cashew butter
- Hemp seed butter
- Macadamia butter
- Peanut butter
- Pecan butter
- Sesame seed butter
- Walnut butter

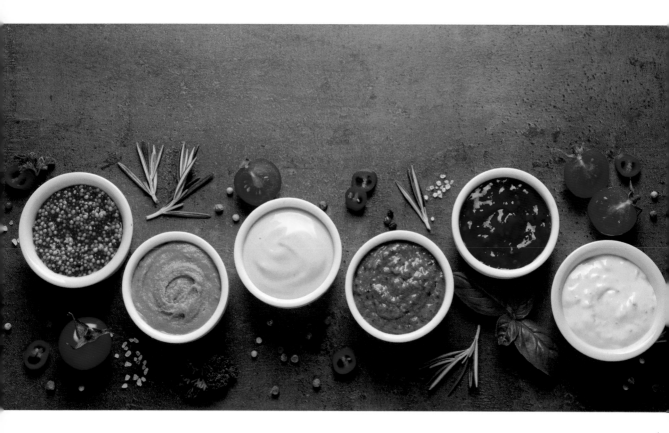

Dressings and Sauces

There are many dressings and sauces that are allowed on the keto nutrition plan. The following premade selections can be found in most grocery stores, but make sure to check the ingredients label to ensure they have no (or very little) sugar. If you prefer to make your own dressings and sauces, please refer to chapter 21.

Wine and Liquor

You can still participate in happy hour or have an adult beverage after a long day of work while on your 30-day keto plan. While some alcoholic drinks are packed with sugar and carbohydrates, others have the proper macros to fit into your nutrition plan if consumed in moderation. Having one (or sometimes two) of the following low-sugar and low-carbohydrate beverages, occasionally, won't sabotage your goals.

Condiments

- Aioli
- Alfredo
- Béarnaise
- Blue cheese dressing
- Buffalo sauce
- Caesar dressing
- Gorgonzola sauce
- Hollandaise
- Hot sauce
- Italian dressing
- Ketchup (sugar-free only)
- Marinara sauce (no added sugars)
- Mayonnaise (avocado oil and regular)
- Mustard
- Pesto
- Ranch dressing
- Soy sauce
- Sriracha
- Tzatziki

Miscellaneous Pantry Items

- Anchovy paste
- Apple cider vinegar
- Balsamic vinegar
- Bouillon cubes
- Broth
- Capers
- Chocolate (at least 75 percent cacao)
- Coconut cream
- Coconut milk (full-fat)
- Curry paste
- Fish sauce
- Red wine vinegar
- Tomato paste (low-carb, sugar-free)
- Vanilla extract

Beverages

- Water
- Sparkling water
- Flavored sparkling water (sugar-free)
- Fruit-infused water (pitcher of water with lemon, lime, cucumber, etc.)
- Unsweetened coffee
- Keto coffee
- Unsweetened tea
- Kombucha (low-sugar only)

Red Wine

- Cabernet sauvignon
- Merlot
- Petite sirah
- Pinot noir
- Syrah
- Zinfandel

White Wine

- Albarino
- Brut champagne
- Chardonnay
- Pinot blanc
- Pinot grigio
- Sauvignon blanc

Liquor*

- Brandy
- Gin
- Rum
- Tequila
- Vodka
- Whisky

*The best keto mixers are club soda, plain sparkling water, and lime juice.

Cooking Oils and Fats			
Type	**Smoke Point**	**Uses**	**Health Benefits**
Olive oil	325–405°F	Low- and medium-heat cooking; "finishing oil" for flavor; salad dressings; marinades; drizzling over lettuces and vegetables.	High in monounsaturated fats, which are linked to lower blood pressure and cholesterol. Consumption linked with improved cognitive health and blood vessel function, and the manufacturing process does not employ chemicals.
Coconut oil	350°F	Roasting at low temperatures, baking, smoothie, shake, or coffee addition. Can be substituted for butter and other oils with a 1:1 ratio.	Provides easily absorbed medium chain fatty acids (MCTs) which are conducive for ketosis. Anti-inflammatory properties and beneficial for gut health.
Medium Chain Triglyceride (MCT) oil	320°F	Used as a supplement and not typically for cooking. Ingredient in salad dressings, smoothies, shakes, and keto coffee.	Higher amount of MCTs than coconut oil—these saturated fats are easily digested and conducive for achieving ketosis. Beneficial for energy and the feeling of satiety.
Avocado oil	520°F	Ideal for grilling, roasting, and panfrying due to high smoke point. Can also be drizzled on salads and vegetables, or as a mayo replacement to add creaminess to dressings, sauces, and dips.	Monounsaturated fat to promote good cholesterol and heart health. Provides vitamin E, antioxidants, and healthy fats.
Walnut oil	320°F	Not ideal for cooking due to low smoke point. Can be added to shakes, smoothies, dressing, sauces, and keto coffee.	Good source of omega-3 fats, which are beneficial for heart, eye, and brain health. The fats found in walnut oil can help to reduce bad cholesterol and increase good cholesterol.
Grass-fed butter	300–350°F	Used for low-heat cooking of eggs, fish, or shellfish. Topper for steak, roasted veggies, or keto chaffles.	Grass-fed butter has a higher composition of omega-3 fatty acids compared to grain-fed butter. Omega-3s are beneficial for heart and brain health, and cholesterol.
Grass-fed ghee	485°F	Used for sautéing meat, poultry, seafood, and vegetables. Can replace butter in most recipes, or be used as a spread.	Ghee is clarified butter, so it is lactose- and casein-free, while still having a buttery taste and texture.

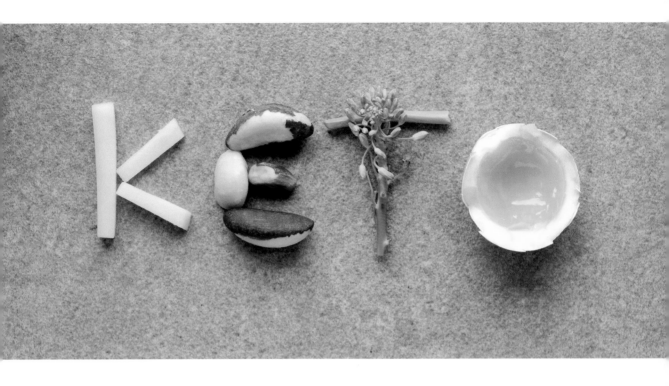

You may be pleasantly surprised that such a large variety of foods is allowed for your 30-day keto plan. And of course, you are not required to use all of these foods, but they are available if you should choose to add them to your grocery cart. Since the list is long and can be overwhelming, we have categorized our favorite (and healthiest!) go-to keto foods in "The Perfect 10 Keto Foods List" on the following pages.

The Perfect 10

As nutritionists, The Perfect 10 is our preferred nutritional foundation for the keto nutrition plan as it promotes not only weight loss but also overall health and wellness. You aren't required to stick solely to the foods found in these ten categories, so feel free to refer back to all listed foods found in this chapter for more variety, as they are all keto-approved. If you aren't familiar with some of the items listed thus far, the recipe chapters found in chapters 18, 19, 20, and 21 will assist you with incorporating many of these foods into a variety of meals and snacks!

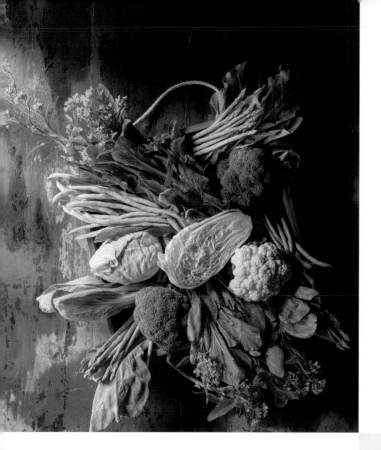

Green Vegetables

Nutrient-dense green vegetables should make up the majority of your 5 percent carbohydrate intake and you can still eat several servings per day while remaining in this general parameter. Nutrient-dense vegetables are low-sugar, unprocessed carbohydrate sources, packed with micronutrients such as thiamine, riboflavin, folate, iron, magnesium, phosphorus, vitamin A, vitamin C, vitamin K, vitamin B6, vitamin C, calcium, potassium, and manganese; they are also chockfull of fiber, which will aid in digestion and regular bowel movements.

Avocado

Avocados have special properties as they are one of the only fatty fruits! Like nutrient-dense vegetables, avocados provide a variety of essential vitamins and minerals, as well as fiber. According to the American Heart Association, the monounsaturated fat found in avocados can help reduce bad cholesterol levels, and the risk of heart attack and stroke. An added benefit, when one consumes fat, is that the brain gets a signal to switch off the appetite. Eating fat slows the breakdown of carbohydrates, which helps keep sugar levels in the blood stable.

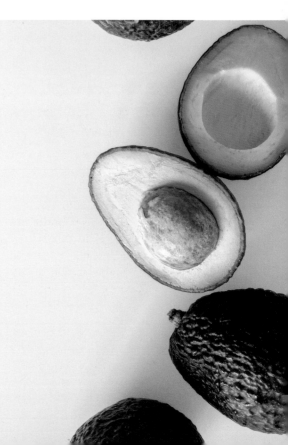

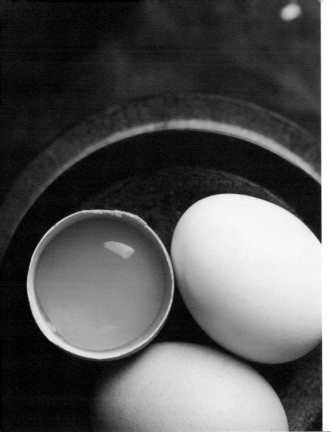

Eggs

Eggs are a nice mix of quality protein and omega-3 fatty acids. Some nutrition and medical circles advise to eat the egg white only, but we urge you to keep that yolk. It is popular belief that the yolk doesn't have any protein, but it does contain 2.7 grams, which is 45 percent of the entire egg's protein composition. The yolk also boasts the superior omega-3 fatty acids, vitamins A, D, E, B12, and K, riboflavin, folate, and iron. Although eggs have been demonized in the past for containing cholesterol, numerous recent studies have cited a general consensus that cholesterol, primarily from egg yolks, poses very little risk for adverse effects on LDL (bad) cholesterol levels.[1]

1   Griffin, BA. "Eggs: Good or Bad?" NCBI. August 1, 2016. Accessed April 6, 2019. ncbi.nlm.nih.gov/pubmed/27126575.

Wild Fatty Fish

In addition to being a source of protein, fatty fish such as wild salmon (if you choose canned salmon, look for "wild Alaskan" on the label) contains omega-3 fatty acids as well. The omega-3 fats found in these types of salmon contain exceptional amounts of the vital DHA and EPA which are the long-chain omega-3s known for being most beneficial for eye, brain, and heart health.[2] In addition to their omega-3 fats, wild salmon contain high amounts of vitamin D, which can be difficult to find in most foods. Another fatty fish that you can get both fresh and canned, mackerel has even lower mercury levels and is at less risk of being overfished.

2   Griffin, B. A. "Eggs: Good or Bad?" NCBI. August 1, 2016. Accessed April 6, 2019. ncbi.nlm.nih.gov/pubmed/27126575.

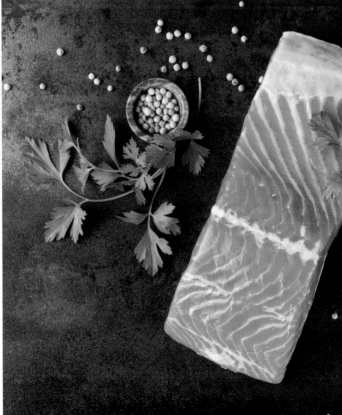

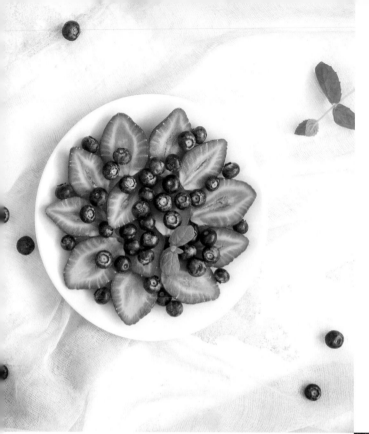

Extremely Low-Sugar Fruits

You can fit a little bit of low-sugar fruit in your keto regimen, but keep in mind your carbohydrate intake should not exceed more than 5 percent of your calories, and many of your allotted carbohydrates will be dedicated to green vegetables. The lowest-sugar fruits are tomato, red bell pepper, olives, and avocado. Olives and avocado are the highest in fat, so those can be consumed much more frequently. Berries are allowed on your plan, but since they are higher in sugar, those will need to be monitored more closely, as too many berries can easily make you exceed your 5 percent carbohydrate limit. Low-sugar fruits do offer essential vitamins, minerals, and fiber, so we definitely recommend eating them, but in true moderation.

Nuts and Seeds

Nuts and seeds are packed with nutrition, providing substantial amounts of good fats, fiber, vitamins, and minerals. Aim to consume a variety of raw nuts and seeds to benefit from a broad spectrum of micronutrients. The nuts and seeds that will pack in the fat without a lot of carbohydrates are macadamia nuts, Brazil nuts, and pecans. Calorie-dense, one ounce as a snack, or used as a topping on a salad, will do!

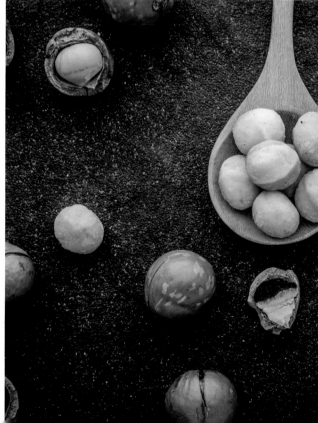

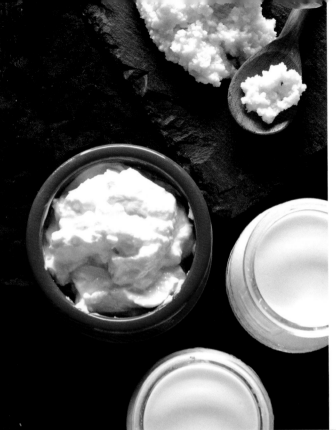

Low-Carbohydrate Probiotic Foods

We all have "good" and "bad" bacteria in our bodies. Probiotics are known as the "friendly bacteria" and consist of *Lactobacillus acidophilus*, *Lactobacillus bulgarius*, *Lactobacillus reuteri*, *Streptococcus thermophiles*, *Saccharomyces boulardii*, *Bifidobacterium bifidum*, and *Bacillus subtilis*. Bad gut bacteria can increase for a variety of reasons (i.e. use of antibiotics, too much alcohol consumption, lack of physical movement, and smoking) so consumption of good bacteria via probiotics is beneficial. Foods that naturally contain probiotics are Greek yogurt, kefir, apple cider vinegar, low-sugar kombucha, dark chocolate, and brine-cured olives. Known as a superior probiotic food, sauerkraut actually does not contain a substantially diverse amount of friendly bacteria, however, its organic acid content supports the growth of good bacteria.

Grass-fed, Organic Red Meat and Organic Poultry

Due to environmental toxins found in many animal proteins, it is ideal to consume organic and/or grass-fed selections if possible (if you choose to consume meat and poultry). When beef, lamb, and venison are grass-fed, the composition of the meat changes, reflecting an Omega-3 fatty acid profile that is more similar to wild salmon. These essential fats contain Docosahexaenoic Acid (DHA) Eicosapentaenoic Acid (EPA). DHA is critical for brain and eye health as it accounts for 40 percent of the polyunsaturated fatty acids found in the brain, and 60 percent found in the retina. Both DHA and EPA are associated with heart and cellular health, as well as lower levels of inflammation. Poultry such as organic turkey and chicken provide B vitamins iron, zinc, potassium, and phosphorus.

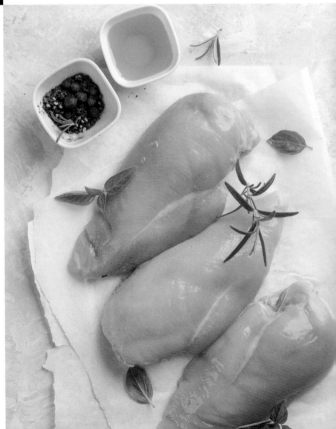

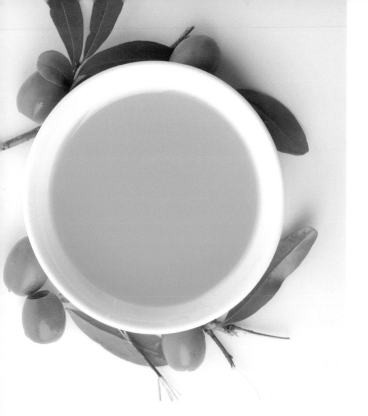

Oils

Oils are a staple of the keto diet, but not all oils are created equally so choosing the highest-quality oils with the most beneficial fat profiles is imperative. In addition, the processing of some oils (such as the use of the neurotoxin hexane for extraction) can have detrimental effects on the quality of the oil, so that is another factor to consider. Some of the best oils for keto, based on fat content and cold-pressed processing, are avocado oil, extra-virgin olive oil, coconut oil, and walnut oil.

Water

Although it's not a food, water does get a spot on "The Perfect 10" as its importance is undeniable. One of the key staples to maintaining proper weight and health is to make good old H2O your primary beverage as it is sugar- and calorie-free. Water assists with dissolving vitamins and minerals, making them more accessible to the body. Also, adequate water intake is essential for the kidneys to function, which will assist with the excretion of waste products.

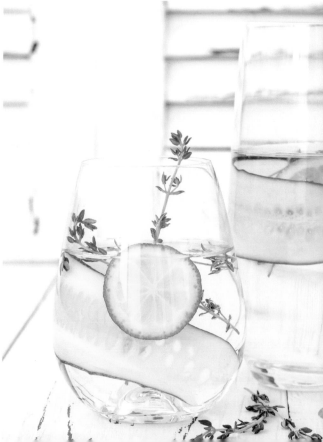

Chapter 5

What You Can't Eat and Why

Since it's easier to avoid the temptation of unhealthy foods when you have concrete evidence as to why they're bad for us, we would like to take some time to explore the reasons why we are eliminating some widely consumed fare. As you have probably noticed, adhering to the 30-day keto plan requires the elimination of many foods, some of which are touted as "healthy" in many circles of the nutrition world (as well as some that should be avoided on any diet), so you may be wondering why those particular items should be avoided. This chapter further explains the reasoning and philosophies behind the keto lifestyle through exploration of foods that should be avoided or limited for weight loss and overall health purposes.

Foods to Eliminate

Bagels
Beans and lentils
Cake
Candy
Cereal
Commercial granola bars
Cookies
Corn
Cow's milk
Crackers
Croissants
Donuts
Fast food and processed foods (even low-carb versions)
Fruit juice and other sugary beverages
Ice cream
Muffins
Pita bread
Pita chips
Pizza crust
Potato chips
Potatoes
Rice
Soda
Tortilla
White bread
White flour
White pasta
Whole wheat bread
Whole wheat flour
Whole wheat pasta

Wheat Products

The majority of the health and nutrition world has concurred that white flour products are potentially weight-adding, empty-calorie foods without much to offer in terms of vitamins and minerals. You may be wondering why whole wheat products are falling into this same category of foods to be eliminated, since they are generally thought of as a healthy requirement of one's diet. More than thirty million Americans (around 10 percent) are afflicted with diabetes, and 90 to 95 percent of these people have type 2 diabetes, which is often caused by diets that include too much sugar. In addition to obvious high-sugar sources such as candy and soda, foods such as whole wheat bread, pasta, cereals, and crackers contain many high-glycemic carbohydrates that will raise blood sugar, and the drastic rise resulting from regular consumption of these foods can lead to type 2 diabetes, cravings, and excessive weight gain. You may still be thinking this couldn't be true for whole wheat foods as the composition of fiber and carbohydrates is drastically different than that of white flour products, however, that simply isn't true. Below is a comparison of whole wheat bread versus white bread and you will see they are extremely similar, the wheat only having a marginal amount of fiber more than the white bread.

	White Bread	**Wheat Bread**
Serving Size	2 pieces (52 grams)	2 pieces (52 grams)
Calories	150	120
Fat	2 grams	1.5 grams
Carbohydrates	28 grams	24 grams
Protein	4 grams	6 grams
Sodium	180 milligrams	220 milligrams
Fiber	1.5 grams	3 grams
Most abundant ingredients per nutrition label	Enriched bleached flour (wheat flour, malted barley flour) water, high-fructose corn syrup	Whole wheat flour, water, high-fructose corn syrup, wheat, gluten, yeast

Besides excessive high-glycemic carbohydrates, another implication of wheat products is that the majority of nonorganic wheat is treated with Roundup which means that a large portion of processed wheat foods also contain glyphosate, a chemical found in the widely used weed killer. According to International Agency for Research on Cancer, glyphosate is classified as a "probable carcinogen." Several studies suggest consuming a "probable carcinogen" is detrimental to our health and even the court system has recently ruled that it can cause unfavorable outcomes such as cancer. Keep in mind that most nonorganic wheat, as well as a multitude of processed foods such as cereals, pastas, and crackers that contain wheat have been treated with glyphosate, so an abundance of wheat products will not only raise blood sugar and cause potential weight gain, but also lead to the excessive consumption of chemicals such as Roundup.

Coincidentally, the majority of foods that contain wheat are also highly processed with a variety of other detrimental ingredients. They have long shelf lives and contain harmful preservatives as well as other additives that will not contribute to your overall health and well-being. Some of these common ingredients that are found in processed wheat foods include but are not limited to soybean oil, high-fructose corn syrup, and soy lecithin.

Like wheat, the majority of US soybeans are treated with Monsanto's glyphosate, therefore the widely popular soybean oil that is found in numerous processed foods is also contaminated with the "probable carcinogen." In addition, a high percentage of US corn is also treated with glyphosate, so not only does high-fructose corn syrup contain a "probable carcinogen," it is also even sweeter than sugar, and we know that excessive sweeteners can contribute to a multitude of health-related ailments. Soy lecithin is an additive that gives food a smooth texture; the chemical solvent hexane (a neurotoxin) is used to extract oil from the soybeans, so traces of hexane will remain in these processed foods. In a nutshell, despite the fact that whole wheat products have been touted for decades as being required for a healthy lifestyle, there is a three-pronged negative with consumption of these products: high-glycemic carbohydrates, relatively low fiber-to-calorie ratio, and traceable amounts of glyphosate/other toxins.

There are some concerns that glyphosate found in Roundup could be correlated with a variety of serious ailments such as celiac disease.[1] Many studies have also indicated that glyphosate exposure may cause DNA damage and cancer in humans.[2] In recent years, a terminally ill California man was awarded $289 million as a result of a jury concluding that glyphosate-containing Roundup caused his non-Hodgkin's lymphoma. The use of the herbicide on genetically modified crops such as corn, soy, and wheat has increased 100-fold since it was introduced in 1974 so further studies may need to be conducted to determine the outcome of this exponentially increased use. To avoid these foods, look for products labeled as "certified organic." Moreover, produce is labeled with PLU (price look-up) codes which are located on the sticker, found on the piece of produce. To guarantee you are not buying a genetically modified food that is likely to have been treated with glyphosate, choose the codes that begin with the number 9—this means the food is organic!

Cow's Milk

The marketing of cow's milk has been quite extensive, leading the masses to believe it is a superior beverage due to its calcium content. Commercial cow's milk contains hormones that are meant for cows, not humans. Even the organic brands of milk contain hormones that are naturally found in the animal, and these estrogens and progesterone may not be ideal for human consumption.[3] In fact, some studies are suggesting that intake of commercial cow's milk may be cause of concern to the general public and more research may be needed.[4]

---

1   Samsel, A., and S. Seneff. "Glyphosate, Pathways to Modern Diseases II: Celiac Sprue and Gluten Intolerance." NCBI. December 2013. Accessed May 11, 2019. nlm.nih.gov/pmc/articles/PMC3945755/.

2   Koller, VJ, M. Furhacker, A. Nersesyan, M. Misik, M. Eisenbauer, and S. Knasmueller. "Cytotoxic and DNA-damaging Properties of Glyphosate and Roundup in Human-derived Buccal Epithelial Cells." NCBI. May 2012. Accessed May 11, 2019. ncbi.nlm.nih.gov/pubmed/22331240.

3   K. Mayurama, T. Oshima, and K. Ohyama, "Exposure to exogenous estrogen through intake of commercial milk produced from pregnant cows.," NCBI, February 2010, accessed September 10, 2017, ncbi.nlm.nih.gov/pubmed/19496976.

4   H. Malekinejad and A. Rezabakhsh, "Hormones in Dairy Foods and Their Impact on Public Health—A Narrative Review Article," June 2015, accessed September 10, 2017, ncbi.nlm.nih.gov/pmc/articles/PMC4524299/.

A rising concern is that modern pregnant cows continue to lactate so they, too, are used in commercial milk production. The milk that comes from pregnant cows have considerably high levels of estrogen and progesterone which are absorbed by one who drinks milk. This hormone absorption is linked with earlier sexual maturation in children as well as lowered levels of testosterone in males.[5] A newer (and ironic) concern is that many studies now show milk consumption may be associated with higher incidence of bone fractures.[6] These are some alarming factors to take into consideration when pondering the common recommendation that you should be consuming three servings of dairy per day to meet your calcium requirements.

When following the 30-day keto plan, keeping sugar intake to a strict minimum is essential to see results, and one cup of cow's milk contains 13 grams of sugar, so following mainstream recommendations of three cups per day would result in 39 grams of sugar just from milk consumption. So, what is one to do? Yes, we need calcium as it is an essential micronutrient especially for bone and heart health, nerve signaling, and muscle function. Fortunately, there are an array of superior nondairy sources of the nutrient, and we will tell you where to find them in coming chapters. In addition, moderate amounts of cheese are keto-approved as the sugar content found in one serving of cheese is typically between zero and one gram. When compared to cheese, Greek yogurt and kefir (a great source of probiotics) tend to be a bit higher in sugar and carbohydrates, so they are allowed on the 30-day keto plan in true moderation (no more than one serving per day).

Starchy Foods

Like breads, pastas, and cereals, other starchy foods such as potatoes, bananas, beans, and rice are not part of the 30-day plan due to high carbohydrate and moderate to high glycemic index rankings (which measures how carbohydrates affect your blood sugar).

---

5   K. Maruyama, T. Oshima, and K. Ohyama, "Exposure to exogenous estrogen through intake of commercial milk produced from pregnant cows.," NCBI, February 2010, accessed September 20, 2017, ncbi.nlm.nih.gov/pubmed/19496976.

6   K. Michaëlsson et al., "Milk intake and risk of mortality and fractures in women and men: cohort studies.," NCBI, October 28, 2014, accessed September 20, 2017, ncbi.nlm.nih.gov/pubmed/25352269.

It's true—there are abundant micronutrients in the potato skin, however, the white filling affects your body in a similar manner to how table sugar does. In fact, in a recent long-term study of 120,000 individuals and the diet patterns that negatively impacted their weights, potatoes were identified as one of the primary culprits that contributed to weight gain.[7] One medium potato has 37 grams of high-glycemic carbohydrates which will create a surge in blood sugar and, as we have mentioned previously, sugar will turn into fat if not burned. We don't want you to miss out on the essential nutrients such as fiber, potassium, vitamin B6, and magnesium that are found in the potato, so you can refer to chapter 13 to see which 30-day keto plan foods boast those particular nutrients.

Rice is another starchy food that is commonly up for debate in nutrition circles. Just like white bread, white rice has been labeled as inferior, while brown rice is consider higher in fiber, and with a lower carbohydrate content. Due to said characteristics of brown rice, it is commonly approved as a weight- and blood-sugar-friendly food. Below is a comparison of white and brown rice so we can examine nutritional profiles of each to find any similarities and differences.

As you can see, the only glaring difference is the fact that the cup of brown rice has roughly three more grams of fiber per cup than the white variety. This one characteristic has

	White Rice	Brown Rice
Serving Size	1 cup	1 cup
Calories	206	216
Fat (grams)	0.4	1.8
Carbohydrates (grams)	45	45
Protein (grams)	4	5
Fiber (grams)	0.6	3.5

been the cause for many nutritionists and doctors to recommend brown rice as a healthy blood sugar and weight-loss tool as the fiber will slow down the digestion of the carbohydrates. The fiber content in the brown rice does make it a better choice, but what many studies do not identify is exactly how much better of a choice it is—some studies suggest that choosing brown rice is an improvement when compared

---

7   Mozaffarian, Dariush, Tao Hao, Eric Rimm, Walter Willett, and Frank Hu. "Changes in Diet and Lifestyle and Long-Term Weight Gain in Women and Men." *New England Journal of Medicine*. June 29, 2011. Accessed April 14, 2019. nejm.org/doi /full/10.1056/NEJMoa1014296.

to white rice, but only a marginal improvement at best. Forty-five grams of carbohydrates in one cup of any food is quite excessive and those three grams of fiber are not going to substantially negate the effects that a food with this nutrition profile has on our blood sugar responses. In fact, some studies have suggested that substituting brown rice for white rice will have no positive effect on those who are at risk for type 2 diabetes.[8] Other studies have suggested that the nutrient profiles in brown rice, despite being superior to white, may have no impact on overall health due to low absorption rates, caused by antinutritional factors present in brown rice.[9] Just like with potatoes, brown rice boasts many essential vitamins and minerals such as fiber, vitamin B6, and magnesium. Chapter 8 will list a variety of foods that contain those nutrients, while having exponentially lesser amounts of carbohydrates, and therefore, more positive effects on your blood sugar and weight maintenance.

Sports Drinks and Fruit Juices

In addition to eating nutrient-dense foods, we recommend staying hydrated, with water as your primary beverage. This can also include unsweetened tea and coffee, as well as unsweetened sparkling water. We highly recommend *against* one of the most common beverage suggestions many receive when trying to lose weight and/or improve overall health, and that faulty advice is to drink sports drinks for hydration and electrolyte replenishment. Popular sports drinks contain a variety of sweeteners such as high-fructose corn syrup and liquefied table sugar, which will not assist your wellness efforts. Even more alarming, some sports drinks contain harmful chemicals such as brominated vegetable oil. Brominated vegetable oil is a combination of bromine and vegetable oil and is similar in composition to brominated flame retardants; this additive is used to

8   Zhang, G., A. Pan, G. Zhong, Z. Yu, H. Wu, X. Chen, L. Tang, Y. Feng, H. Zhou, H. Li, B. Hong, WC Willett, VS Malik, D. Spiegelman, FB Hu, and X. Lin. "Substituting White Rice with Brown Rice for 16 Weeks Does Not Substantially Affect Metabolic Risk Factors in Middle-aged Chinese Men and Women with Diabetes or a High Risk for Diabetes." NCBI. September 01, 2011. Accessed April 14, 2019. ncbi.nlm.nih.gov/pubmed/21795429.

9   Callegaro, D., and J. Tirapegui. "[Comparison of the Nutritional Value between Brown Rice and White Rice]." NCBI. October/November 1996. Accessed April 14, 2019. ncbi.nlm.nih.gov/pubmed/9302338.

remove any cloudiness to the appearance of the beverage. Banned in the Japan and Europe, consumption of brominated vegetable oil is associated with thyroid disease, memory loss, fatigue, tremors, skin rashes, cancer, and hormone disorders.

Sports drinks are commonly suggested for electrolyte replacement, however, the risks of consuming these sports drinks for electrolytes outweigh the benefits. Electrolytes are minerals such as calcium, potassium, sodium, and magnesium, and we do excrete this through bodily fluids, so yes, it is important to replenish these minerals. You can do so by eating mineral-containing foods including but not limited to vegetables, low-sugar fruits, fish, and meats.

You may be curious about fruit juices, given the fact that some mainstream advice suggests that sugar from fruit is natural and therefore, can be consumed quite freely, without consequence. Unfortunately, the sugar from fruit (fructose) impacts our blood sugar in a similar manner than table sugar does, therefore excessive sugar consumption from fruits and fruit juices is not keto-approved. Fruit juices are merely concentrated versions of the fruit itself, and you can see the sugar implications below when we take several pieces of fruit and condense them into one cup of juice. Not to mention, the commercial processing of juice strips the fiber content that is naturally found in the fruit. Below you will see the comparison of sugar and fiber found in one piece of fruit versus a cup of the corresponding fruit's juice.

	Calories	Sugar (grams)	Fiber (grams)
1 orange	45	9	2.3
Orange juice (1 cup)	111	21	0.5
1 apple	78	15	3.6
Apple juice (1 cup)	113	24	0.5
½ large grapefruit	52	8	2
Grapefruit juice (1 cup)	96	18	0.2

Artificial Sweeteners

Artificial sweeteners add sweetness to foods without adding calories. Some keto circles approve the use of aspartame (Equal or NutraSweet), acesulfame potassium (Sunett), and sucralose (Splenda) to give more flavor without impacting weight gain or blood sugar levels. Studies are now suggesting that regular consumption of artificial sweeteners in the general population are actually associated with negative health outcomes such as type 2 diabetes and metabolic disorders, as opposed to helping prevent them.[10] Not to mention, certain artificial sweeteners such as aspartame are associated with cancer risks due carcinogenic properties.[11] Moderate use of stevia is approved in some keto circles as it is a zero-calorie sweetener that is derived from the plant species *Stevia rebaudiana*, native to Brazil and Paraguay. Although it is easier said than done, training your taste buds to not crave added sweeteners to beverages and foods is a key outcome we would like you to achieve from your 30-day keto plan.

Processed Meats

Salami, bacon, hot dogs, sausage, and cold cuts fit into the protein and fat categories of traditional keto nutrition plans, so you may be wondering why you are finding them in this chapter of what not to eat. We aren't saying you have to eliminate these foods altogether, but we do advise to eat no more than two to three servings of these foods per week, despite the fact they do assist with meeting your macronutrient requirements. The primary reason why we advise to limit consumption of these items if because they are very high in sodium and contain detrimental additives such as potentially carcinogenic nitrates, as well as butylated hydroxytoluene (BHT), and butylated hydroxyanisole (BHA), both of which increase shelf life (for a thorough examination of additives such as BHT and BHA, please refer to chapter 15). The regular consumption of additives found

10 S. Swithers, "Artificial sweeteners produce the counterintuitive effect of inducing metabolic derangements," NCBI, September 2013, accessed September 24, 2017, ncbi.nlm.nih.gov/pmc/articles/PMC3772345/.

11 Soffritti, M., M. Padovani, E. Tibaldi, L. Falcioni, F. Manservisi, and F. Belpoggi. "The Carcinogenic Effects of Aspartame: The Urgent Need for Regulatory Re-evaluation." NCBI. April 2014. Accessed April 14, 2019. ncbi.nlm.nih.gov/pubmed/24436139.

in processed meats have been associated with colorectal cancer, which is the first cause of cancer death of nonsmokers in affluent countries.[12]

Fast Food and Processed Foods

Fast-food meals are known to be loaded with empty calories, high-glycemic carbohydrates, sugar, and bad fats, but that is just the tip of the iceberg. If you order the typical burger, fries, and a soft drink at a fast-food establishment, you are likely to consume a combination of butylated hydroxyanisole, trans-fatty acids, dimethylpolysiloxane, and azodicarbonamide. If you have never heard of some of these ingredients and are unaware of their implications, you are not alone. These items are lurking in the majority of all fast-food items and have serious consequences for our health. Since we are trying to achieve overall health and wellness, fast foods and processed foods are not allowed on the 30-day plan since most contain the following additives.

Butylated Hydroxyanisole

Butylated Hydroxyanisole (BHA) is a chemical food additive put in oils so the oils can be used multiple times without going rancid. BHA is a known carcinogen, and several studies have shown links between the chemical and cancerous tumors in animals, as well as stomach cancer in humans. Many fast-food baked goods, fried foods, dehydrated potatoes, and meat products contain butylated hydroxyanisole.

Trans-Fatty Acids

Trans-fatty acids (or trans fats) are created by adding hydrogen to vegetable oil; many fast food establishments use this type of fat because it is cheap and has a longer shelf life compared to other fats. When using this type of oil in deep fryers, it doesn't have to be changed as often since it takes longer to spoil. Trans fats are known for raising your LDL (bad) cholesterol while lowering your HDL (good) cholesterol. Animal studies

---

12 Santarelli, RL, F. Pierre, and D. Corpet. "Processed Meat and Colorectal Cancer: A Review of Epidemiologic and Experimental Evidence." NCBI. March 25, 2008. Accessed April 14, 2019. ncbi.nlm.nih.gov/pmc/articles/PMC2661797/.

have shown that regular consumption of trans-fatty acids has led to memory difficulties, amplified emotional reactions, and oxidative injury in the brain cells of animals.[13]

Hydrolyzed Vegetable Proteins

Vegetable protein—it doesn't sound so bad? Hydrolyzed vegetable proteins are created when foods such as soy, corn, and wheat are boiled in hydrochloric acid and neutralized with sodium hydroxide, which breaks the proteins in the vegetables down into amino acids. Monosodium glutamate (MSG) is one of the amino acids. One of the most widely used food additives, MSG is regarded as "safe" in moderation by many popular websites and sources, however, research has linked it to obesity, metabolic disorders, neurotoxic effects, and detrimental effects on reproductive organs.[14]

Dyes and Artificial Flavors

Dyes and artificial flavors are used by many fast-food establishments and commercial food manufacturers to replace real food by providing fake color and flavor to menu items. Brightly colored desserts, sodas, and macaroni and cheese contain dyes that are prospective carcinogens such as Yellow No. 5 and No. 6. Some countries, including England, require labeling of products that contain Yellow No. 5 and No. 6 as it has been linked to hyperactivity in children. The United States has banned some dyes, however, Blue No. 1, Blue No. 2, Green No. 3, Red No. 3, Red No. 40, Yellow No. 5, and Yellow No. 6 still remain on the FDA's approved list—yet another reason to check your ingredients labels!

Dimethylpolysiloxane

Dimethylpolysiloxane is derived from silicon and is found in hair and skin conditioners, cosmetics, and Silly Putty. It is used in cooking oils as an anti-foaming agent to prevent

13   CS Pase et al., "Influence of perinatal trans fat on behavioral responses and brain oxidative status of adolescent rats acutely exposed to stress.," NCBI, September 5, 2013, accessed September 2, 2017, ncbi.nlm.nih.gov/pubmed/23742847.

14   Niaz, K., E. Zaplatic, and J. Spoor. "Extensive Use of Monosodium Glutamate: A Threat to Public Health?" NCBI. March 19, 2018. Accessed May 11, 2019. ncbi.nlm.nih.gov/pmc/articles/PMC5938543/.

spattering oil, and is found in items like chicken nuggets, French fries, and fried sand-wiches. In addition, it even lurks in fountain drinks to limit excess foam you typically get with canned and bottled sodas. Dimethylpolysiloxane is used in a wide variety of fast-food establishments, including ones that claim to use higher-quality, healthier, and even organic ingredients.

Azodicarbonamide

One of the more recently controversial food additives as it is also used in yoga mats, azo-dicarbonamide (ADA) is a flour bleaching agent and dough conditioner that is banned in most of Europe, as well as Australia and Singapore. Considered to be a carcinogen, ADA is linked to cancer, neurological disorders, cell mutations, and disrupted hormone functions in animals. Many fast-food and commercial food manufacturers have eliminated this ingredient from their products, but it still remains in a variety of processed foods.

Making the best food choices for yourself and your family can be hard some-times—especially when there are so many hidden ingredients in our food supply! Of course, fast food and processed foods can be delicious (since they are purposely formulated to be that way!) so when one is aware of the implications of the hidden ingredients, these foods may be easier to resist. Once your healthiest keto habits are firmly established upon completing your 30-day keto plan, very occasional low-carbohydrate and low-sugar fast food can be eaten, if you're in a bind and need something quick.

Chapter 6

You Have Questions, We Have Answers

If you have questions about your 30-day keto plan, you will probably find the answers in this chapter. Essentially, you can consider the answers to these questions as rules to follow during your 30-day keto plan and yes, some of the "rules" may sound a little strict, but just remember, you can do anything for thirty days. After you complete your 30-day keto plan, you will see incredible results and your relationship with food will be drastically changed. Those who complete this plan realize they may have previously been consuming excessive amounts of sugar, carbohydrates, and processed foods. Improvements in how you feel and the noticeable changes in your body will convince you to not resort back to the standard American diet of excessive amounts of sugar, breads, pastas, cereals, crackers, and processed foods. These rules are in place to help take the guesswork out of your eating plan for the next month, and you will also find solutions to common roadblocks.

In a quick summary, what can and can't I eat during my 30-day keto plan?
You can and should eat low-carbohydrate vegetables, extremely low-sugar fruits, seafood, meat, poultry, eggs, cheese, cottage cheese, Greek yogurt, cream, butter, ghee, nuts, seeds, oils, dark chocolate, and keto-approved condiments such as mayonnaise, dressings, and sauces. You cannot consume bread, cereal, pasta, rice, crackers, potatoes, low-fat dairy, moderate- or high-carbohydrate fruits and vegetables, starches, sugary foods, soda, fruit juice, and typical dessert foods.

What are macronutrients and why are they important to know about?

Fats, carbohydrates, and proteins are the three macronutrients found in the diet. For keto, fat intake should be between 70 and 80 percent of total calories, carbohydrate intake should be between 5 and 10 percent of total calories, and protein should be between 10 and 20 percent of total calories.

How many grams of carbohydrates should I have per day?

This is a tricky question since we are all different, so carbohydrate amounts will vary from person to person. Generally speaking, you should stick to 50 grams of total carbohydrates or less per day, or 25 grams of net carbohydrates (total carbohydrates minus grams of fiber) or less per day.

How do I track all of my carbohydrates, fats, and proteins?

There are many online macro tracking apps that are simple to use—one of the most popular ones in the keto community is called Carb Manager. If you're worried about this being too much work, it will only last two to three weeks before you naturally are accustomed to knowing what foods have the proper amount of carbohydrates, fats, and proteins for your nutrition plan. Although this process may seem daunting in the beginning, it gets much easier, and before you know it, you won't need to track anymore as you will know what is in most foods.

Do I need to track my calories, too?

People of different heights, weights, ages, activity levels, and goals all have assorted calorie requirements. Not to mention, when it comes to weight loss, calories in versus calories expended will always matter to some degree. Even if you hit your macro requirements in perfect ranges, you could still fail to lose weight (or even gain weight) if you overeat too many calories. There are several online tools to help you determine how many calories you should consume to maintain or lose weight.

Will the keto diet make my cholesterol worse since it's high in fat?

One of the primary guidelines of the 30-day keto plan is to choose the healthiest fats possible. Fats found in foods such as avocado, extra-virgin olive oil, nuts, seeds, and wild salmon actually help promote good cholesterol. If one focuses on unhealthy fats such as inferior oils and processed meats, then it is possible that negative outcomes such as increased bad cholesterol and excessive sodium levels could occur. There are several studies showing that the ketogenic nutrition plan is associated with improvements in good cholesterol, cardiovascular risk, and type 2 diabetes.[1]

Will I get enough fiber and micronutrients?

If your 5 to 10 percent allotted carbohydrates are dedicated to mostly green vegetables and low-sugar fruits, you can get the required fiber, vitamin, and mineral intake. The average American only consumes 10 to 15 grams of fiber per day, so if you plan correctly, you can double the amount of fiber that the average person gets if you watch what you eat. The table below illustrates one example (there are several other combinations in which you can achieve this with different produce) of how you can get 24 grams of fiber while remaining under your limit of 25 grams of net carbohydrates. Not to mention, the consumption of this many servings of low-sugar produce will give a substantial amount of essential vitamins, minerals, and antioxidants.

Food	Net Carbohydrates (grams)	Fiber (grams)
1 cup cooked spinach	2	4
2 cups chopped romaine	1	2
2 cups cooked broccoli	12	10
½ cup raspberries	7	8
Totals	**22 grams**	**24 grams**

---

1   Kosinski, Christophe, and François R Jornayvaz. "Effects of Ketogenic Diets on Cardiovascular Risk Factors: Evidence from Animal and Human Studies." *Nutrients*. MDPI, May 19, 2017. ncbi.nlm.nih.gov/pmc/articles/PMC5452247/.

Will I have to spend a lot of time cooking?

Typically speaking, some cooking and food preparation does come along with the territory of living a healthy lifestyle. To complete the 30-day keto plan, you will need to spend an average of three hours per week (or twenty-five minutes per day) in the kitchen. Of course, it could be done in less time if you are one who eats in restaurants frequently (refer to chapter 9 for your guide to restaurant keto).

So I can eat in restaurants during my 30-day plan? Can I get fast food, too?

Some who are looking to lose weight or improve health are reluctant to even try a keto nutrition plan as they assume restaurants will be off limits. Let's face it, a large percentage of the population eat in restaurants on a regular basis due to work obligations, social gatherings, and just for plain convenience. We have dedicated a chapter for those who fall into this category, however, fast food *is not allowed* on your 30-day keto plan. We are looking to optimize health and well-being, and fast food is packed with low-quality fats and proteins, sodium, chemicals, and other additives (examined in chapter 5) that are not conducive to health and wellness. After your 30-day plan, you can add occasional fast food back in, in moderation, while following the restaurant and food swap guidelines.

Can I eat any sort of fat to fulfill my 70 to 80 percent fat requirement?

During your 30-day keto plan, we urge against a "free-for-all" of consuming any and all fats just for the sake the fulfilling your macronutrient quotas. Most people do not consume enough omega-3 fatty acids, because only certain foods contain them. Omega-3 fats are not produced by our bodies, so we need to get them from our diet; they assist with brain function, heart health, and reducing inflammation. Good fats also help our blood sugar levels to remain even and they can help us feel full for longer. Some examples of foods that have the healthiest fats are oysters, egg yolks, salmon, mackerel, grass-fed beef, avocado oil, olive oil, walnuts, macadamia nuts, chia seeds, and avocado.

I always eat things like sandwiches and cereal—what will I replace those items with?

There are many common mainstream foods that are a part of standard diets, but they are not allowed on the keto nutrition plan due to higher carbohydrate and sugar content. This table of simple keto food swaps will help you navigate the best and tastiest substitutions.

Instead of This	Have This
Cheeseburger on a bun	Cheeseburger with no bun, or wrapped in lettuce
Sandwich on bread	Sandwich fillings wrapped in lettuce or over a bed of greens
Chicken pasta dish	Chicken with riced cauliflower or zucchini noodles and sauce
Steak with potatoes	Steak with vegetables or salad
Sugary salad with cranberries, candied nuts, and sweet dressing	Salad with nuts, cheese, avocado, protein, and savory oil-based dressing
Sides like French fries, rice, potato, bread, or pasta	Extra vegetables topped with butter or oil, mashed or riced cauliflower, small side salad topped with oil-based dressing
Chicken fingers or other breaded proteins with ketchup	Grilled chicken or other grilled proteins with creamy dipping sauce such as avocado oil mayo
Tacos in tortillas	Lettuce-wrapped tacos
Burritos in tortillas	Burrito bowls with protein, vegetables, cheese, avocado, sour cream, and salsa—no rice or beans
Piece of toast with peanut butter	Celery sticks with peanut butter
Ice cream	Berries topped with heavy whipping cream
Bread basket	Charcuterie board with cheese, meats, olives, and nuts
Dessert of cookies or baked goods	Red wine with dark chocolate and cheese
Standard breakfast of omelet, bacon, potatoes, and toast	Omelet with cheese, bacon, and sliced tomatoes or berries
Sweetened coffee beverage	Unsweetened coffee with coconut oil, cream, butter, or MCT oil
Salted chips	Salted nuts

Can I use artificial sweeteners or keto-approved sweeteners?

No forms of sweeteners are allowed—but it's only for thirty days! You can do it! It may be obvious not to add sugar, however, you also may not use sugar substitutes that are keto-approved in some circles. Kicking a sugar habit means training your taste buds (yes, they are trainable!) to not feel the need to sweeten food and drinks. This can be difficult as we have discussed how the standard American diet tends to make us sugar addicted, but it is possible to break the habit and ridding sugar and sugar substitutes from your life for thirty days will help make the transition to living a lower-sugar lifestyle.

Do I have to pack my food?

Packing a healthy lunch or at least some healthy snacks to have around the office or at school is one of the most efficient ways to combat workplace donuts and vending machines because if you're not hungry, passing up the treats is far easier. We don't want you spending hours in your kitchen, so please refer to chapter 10 to learn how to batch cook.

Do I have to buy organic produce, grass-fed meats and butter, and wild fish to do keto?

No, you do not. We recommend these options since they help limit pesticides and environmental toxins, however, sometimes they are not readily available and they can be expensive. You can still adhere to your 30-day keto plan even if you choose conventional versions of these foods.

Do I have to measure ketones to make sure I'm in ketosis?

No, you are not required to do this. Some find it helpful, however, a large percentage of keto dieters do not take this extra step. You may see dramatic weight loss and blood sugar level improvements just by following the keto nutrition protocol as your sugar and carbohydrate intake will be drastically cut. That alone is typically effective for results.

If I cave and eat something sugary or with lots of carbohydrates, do I have to quit and start over with my 30 days?

No! Jump back on that wagon immediately! Many popular diets require one to start over if a piece (or even a bite) of cake at a birthday party occurs. This train of thought can lead to reluctance and even anxiety when it comes to taking the first step to making a lifestyle change. There is misconception that proper nutrition has to be followed 100 percent of the time and there is no wiggle room if you want to see results, but that can't be further from the truth. You will see progress (and lots of it) if you adhere to the keto principles and strategies *most of the time*. There may be situations when a slipup occurs—acknowledge it, don't feel guilty about it, and jump right back on the wagon.

Can I use processed and packaged foods that say they are keto-approved?

No. Your 30-day keto plan is a break from sugar, fast food, and processed foods—it's a reset to give perspective on how many of these items we may have been consuming in the past. We are aiming for wellness (not just weight loss), and one of the most effective ways in achieving good health is by eating unprocessed foods that come from nature. Here is an example laundry list of hard-to-pronounce ingredients found in one popular keto brand processed snack: soy protein concentrate, medium chain triglycerides, tapioca starch, water, 3-hydroxy butyric acid calcium salt, soy fiber, 3-hydroxy butyric acid sodium salt, 3-hydroxy butyric acid potassium salt, 3-hydroxy butyric acid magnesium monohydrate, sodium caseinate, beet juice powder (color), natural flavors, salt, potato starch and dehydrated potato, sea salt, tomato powder, dehydrated onion, sunflower oil, sunflower lecithin, sodium diacetate, paprika extract, malic acid, citric acid, dehydrated garlic, sodium caseinate (milk), yeast extract, yeast torula, sodium gluconate, potassium chloride, acacia gum, spice extracts, turmeric extract, spices.

The ketogenic diet can seem daunting and hard to understand—we hope this "Q and A" chapter has cleared up any confusion. Like any nutrition lifestyle, once you sort out the facts and get into a routine, you'll find that keto is pretty simple. Once you complete your 30-day keto plan, you'll be so well-versed that the days of tracking macronutrients or searching for questions and answers will be over!

Chapter 7

Intro to Batch Cooking—
Nine Days of Meals

We hope the first few days (or more!) of your 30-day keto plan went well and that you're already seeing and/or feeling some results! This chapter gradually introduces you to batch cooking, where you'll make three days' worth of breakfasts and lunches ahead of time so you have them on hand for your busy schedule of work, school, and family. You will find three meal plan options accompanied with corresponding grocery lists. If you're already in your own groove by using the Keto Meal Planning Kit from the first two days (see page 3 for a refresher), you can stick with it, or if you prefer to prepare meals ahead of time (since that cuts down on preparation and grocery shopping time) for the next three days, this chapter is for you.

Food Storage Containers

Compartmentalized "bento" boxes are quite popular for organized food preparation, but any regular square/rectangular glass or plastic storage containers will work just as well. Jars are also commonly used for salads and parfaits, but your preferred containers will do.

You will be preparing one breakfast and one lunch to take with you for your day at work and/or school so we do recommend having at least two sets for each of those daily meals. Many prefer to have at least six sets to batch cook and store six meals (three breakfasts and three lunches) at a time. If you prefer to only purchase two sets (one for lunch and one for breakfast), you can easily rinse them out each evening and replate your previously batch-cooked food again in the same meal storage containers. Snacks can simply be taken in plastic or reusable bags.

A Note About Repetition

Yes, you will be eating some of the same foods in the coming weeks because extremely varied meal plans call for lots of grocery shopping, meaning more time and money spent. If you're someone who likes more variety, refer to the meal planning system in chapter 14, or if you want to get even more creative in the kitchen, simply choose breakfast, lunch, and dinner recipes from chapters 18, 19, and 20. Typically, for a 30-day keto plan that will kick-start your progress, we advise to make your food prep as simple (and fast) as possible so you don't burn out and can quickly learn the ropes. This chapter provides examples, though you can always design your own batch-cooking plans, with the following as a guide.

The following three-day grocery list and meal plan options are designed for ease of shopping and prepping, while achieving continued results for the next 72 hours. Keep in mind, you can make reasonable substitutions. For example, chicken and ground beef are less expensive options, compared to steak and salmon. You can make protein substitutions based on your own taste and cost preferences. Moreover, if you don't like a particular vegetable in the lists, you can substitute those as well. For a complete list of allowed foods, refer back to chapter 4 to ensure you are making keto-approved replacements.

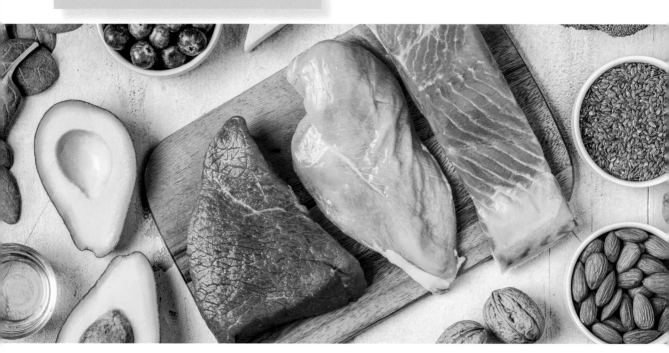

Breakfast and Lunch Meal Prep Grocery List: Option 1

Breakfast Omelet Mugs

1 dozen eggs $3.99

1 large yellow onion $1.00

1 bunch green onions $1.00

1 package shredded cheese $3.99

1 package bacon (optional) $2.99

Chicken and Greek Salad Lunch Boxes

3 chicken breasts $8.99

1 head broccoli $1.99

1 red onion $1.00

1 large cucumber $1.00

1 small carton grape tomatoes $2.99

1 small jar olives $3.99

1 small package feta cheese $3.99

Salt and pepper, to taste

Creamy Taco Soup Dinners

1 pound ground beef $4.99

Yellow onion (purchased for breakfast) $0.00

1 small package garlic cloves $1.99

1 small green bell pepper $1.00

1 (10-ounce) can tomatoes $1.00

1 (8-ounce) package cream cheese $1.99

1 packet taco seasoning (low-sugar) $1.00

1 (14.5-ounce) can beef broth $1.99

1 avocado $1.00

Shredded cheese (purchased for breakfast) $0.00

Total Cost: $51.88

Average Cost Per Meal: $5.76

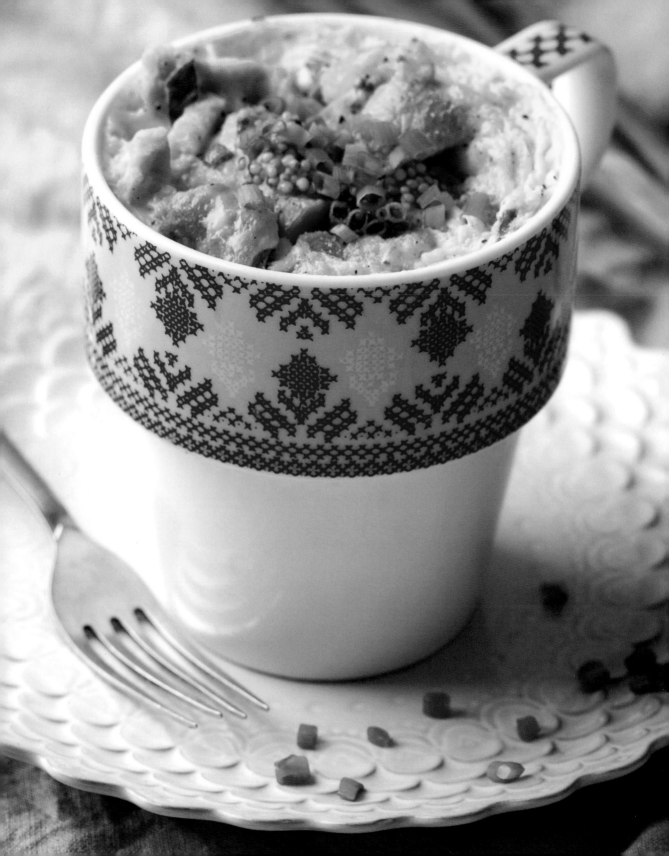

Breakfast Omelet Mugs

Serves 1 for 3 days

Ingredients:

3 tablespoons butter

6–9 whole eggs

3 tablespoons finely chopped yellow onion

3 green onions, finely chopped

6 tablespoons shredded cheese

6 slices cooked bacon, crumbled (optional)

Steps:

1. Beat all ingredients together until thoroughly combined.

2. Divide into 3 equal parts and pour into 3 separate plastic zip-top bags, and place in refrigerator until ready to use.

3. To prepare, pour one omelet mixture into a coffee mug and microwave on high heat for 1 minute.

4. Remove from the microwave and beat again with a fork to combine the partially cooked eggs.

5. Place in the microwave for 30 more seconds and enjoy.

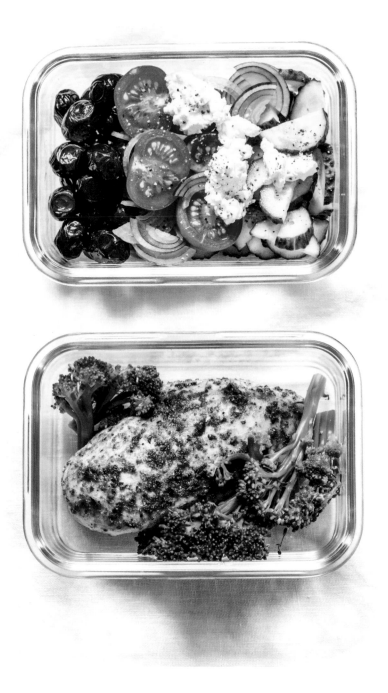

Chicken and Greek Salad Lunch Boxes

Serves 1 for 3 days

Ingredients:

3 chicken breasts
2 tablespoons oil
Your favorite seasonings
1 head broccoli, chopped
    into florets
1 red onion, thinly sliced
1 large cucumber, thinly
    sliced
9 grape tomatoes, halved
20 olives
1 cup feta cheese, crumbled
Oil and vinegar for serving

Steps:

1. In a large pan over medium-high heat, cook the chicken breasts in oil and your favorite seasonings for 3 minutes until browned on one side. Flip the chicken over and reduce heat to medium and cover. Continue to cook until you have reached an internal temperature of 170°F, around 12 to 15 minutes, depending on thickness of chicken.

2. Meanwhile, steam the broccoli florets until tender, around 18 minutes.

3. While the chicken and broccoli are cooking, place the onion, cucumber, tomatoes, and olives in a medium bowl and combine.

4. Divide into 3 equal parts and place into separate meal containers. Top each salad with ⅓ cup feta cheese.

5. Divide the broccoli into thirds and place into the meal containers, followed by one chicken breast in each meal container.

6. Store in the refrigerator and top salad with oil and vinegar before serving.

Creamy Taco Soup Dinner

Serves 1 for 3 days

Ingredients:

1 tablespoon oil

1 pound ground beef (or turkey or chicken)

1 small onion, diced

2–3 cloves garlic, minced

1 small green bell pepper, diced

10 ounces canned tomatoes (or 1 large tomato, chopped)

8 ounces cream cheese

1 packet low-sugar taco seasoning

Salt and pepper to taste

1½ cups beef broth

1 avocado (for serving)

Shredded cheese (for serving)

Steps:

1. Add oil to a large pot and brown the beef, onion, and garlic over medium-high heat for 7 to 8 minutes or until the ground beef is browned through.

2. Add the bell pepper, tomatoes, cream cheese, and spices. Stir for 4 to 5 minutes or until tomatoes are soft and tender and cream cheese is mixed through.

3. Pour in beef broth and reduce heat to low-medium. Simmer 15 to 20 minutes or until desired thickness is achieved.

4. Divide soup into 3 meal containers and store in the refrigerator. To serve, reheat in the microwave and top with sliced avocado and shredded cheese.

Breakfast and Lunch Meal Prep Grocery List: Option 2

Keto Parfait Breakfast Cups

20 ounces full-fat coconut milk or full-fat cottage cheese $3.99

1 carton raspberries (or other berries) $2.99

1 small package chia seeds (optional) $4.99

Tuna Niçoise Lunch Jars

15–20 ounce package of raw spinach or other greens $2.99

3 cans tuna packed in water $5.99

3 hard-boiled eggs $0.75

1 jar olives $2.99

1 package green beans $1.99

2 small tomatoes $1.00

2x Dinner Options

1 pound chicken breast $5.99

1 package shredded cheese $3.99

1 jar chunky salsa $1.99

1 avocado $1.00

1 small container sour cream $1.00

1 (6–8 ounce) steak $8.99

Green beans (already purchased for lunch) $0.00

Total Cost: $50.64
Average Cost Per Meal: $5.62

Keto Parfait Breakfast Cups

Serves 1 for 3 days

Ingredients:

20 ounces full-fat coconut milk or full-fat cottage cheese, divided

3 tablespoons chia seeds, divided

Vanilla extract, to taste (optional)

1 small carton berries of choice

Steps:

1. Divide the coconut milk or cottage cheese between 3 separate jars or other food storage containers and mix 1 tablespoon chia seeds into each jar.

2. Add a dash of vanilla to the mixture and combine (optional).

3. Top each with your berries—4 to 6 sliced strawberries, a small handful of raspberries or blueberries, etc.—and store in the refrigerator until ready to eat.

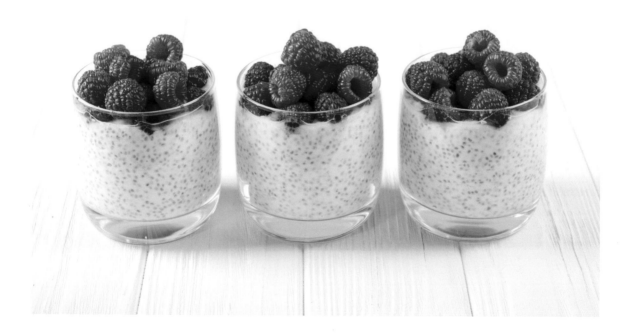

Tuna Niçoise Lunch Jars

Serves 1 for 3 days

Ingredients:

3 cans tuna packed in water

2 small tomatoes, diced

15–20 ounces raw spinach or your favorite greens, chopped

20 green beans, steamed or sautéed and chopped

3 hard-boiled eggs, halved

15 whole olives

Oil, vinegar, and freshly squeezed lemon juice for topping

Steps:

1. Drain the cans of tuna and divide one each into the bottom of each of the 3 jars.

2. Evenly divide the diced tomatoes and place on top of the tuna.

3. Place 1 cup spinach or lettuce on top of the tomatoes in all 3 jars.

4. Divide the green beans into 3 equal parts and place on the lettuce.

5. Add 2 egg halves to each jar.

6. Top with 5 olives each.

7. Before eating, top with oil, vinegar, and freshly squeezed lemon; close the lid and shake to evenly distribute the dressing.

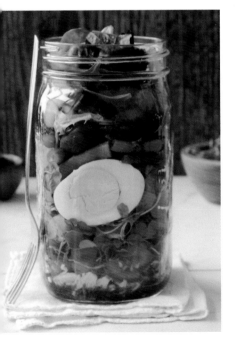

Dinner Option 1:
Cheesy Salsa Chicken

Serves 1 for 2 dinners

Ingredients:

Oil
½ pound chicken breast, cubed
2-3 tablespoons salsa
⅓ cup shredded cheese
½ avocado, sliced
Sour cream, to taste

Steps:

1. Using oil, pan cook the chicken over medium-high heat until almost cooked through, around 10 minutes. (This chicken will be used for two dinners, so you can cook the entire pound of cubed chicken and set half aside before step 2 and refrigerate.)
2. Add the salsa and toss to heat the salsa, around 1 minute.
3. Add shredded cheese and cook until melted, around 1 minute.
4. Plate and top with any excess salsa or cheese that may be left in the pan.
5. Serve with sliced avocado and sour cream.

Dinner Option 2:
Steak and Buttered Green Beans

Serves 1 for 1 dinner

Ingredients:

Seasonings
1 (6-8 ounce) steak
1 tablespoon butter or ghee
7-12 whole green beans

Steps:

1. Preheat a medium pan over high heat, season your steak to your preference, and then place in the hot pan.
2. After 1 minute of sizzling, lower to medium heat and then flip the steak over after 4 minutes.
3. Meanwhile, in a small pan, heat the butter or ghee (you can use oil if you prefer) over medium-low heat and toss in the green beans and season. Cover and continue to cook until tender (around 8 minutes), flipping occasionally to prevent burning.
4. Continue to cook the steak until you have reached an internal temperature of 155°F for medium or 165°F for well done.
5. Plate the steak and green beans, and serve warm.

Breakfast and Lunch Meal Prep Grocery List and Meal Plan: Option 3

Breakfast Charcuterie Boxes

½ dozen eggs $1.99

1 bunch asparagus $3.99

1 (8-ounce) package smoked salmon $7.99

1 package sliced cheese $3.99

1 package of almonds, pecans, or pistachios $5.99

Roasted Chicken and Veggie Lunch Boxes

1 package broccoli florets $1.99

1 red onion $1.00

1 bell pepper $1.00

1½ pounds chicken breast $6.99

Nuts (purchased for breakfast) $0.00

2x Dinner Options

1 pound ground beef $4.99

2 slices cheese (purchased for breakfast) $0.00

1 small zucchini $1.00

1 (6–8 ounce) salmon fillet $7.99

1 package brussels sprouts $2.99

1 small head cauliflower $1.99

1 package grated Parmesan cheese $3.99

Total Cost: $57.88

Average Cost Per Meal $6.43

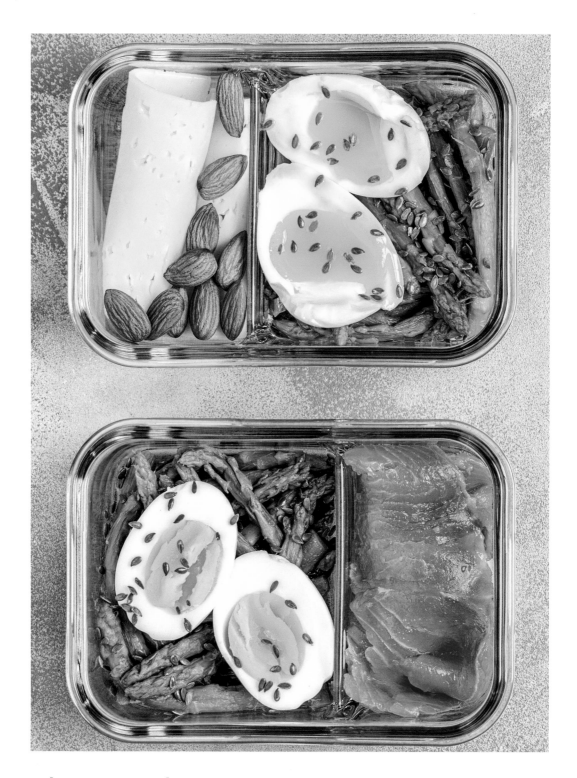

Breakfast Charcuterie Boxes

Serves 1 for 3 days

Ingredients:

6 whole eggs
1 bunch asparagus
Oil
Seasonings
6–8 ounces smoked salmon
3–6 slices cheese
3 ounces almonds, pecans,
  or pistachios

Steps:

1. In a medium pot of boiling water, soft-boil six eggs for 8 to 9 minutes or hard-boil for 11 to 12 minutes.

2. While the eggs are boiling, pan sauté the asparagus using oil and your favorite seasonings until tender, around 5 to 8 minutes depending on thickness.

3. Once the eggs are done boiling to your liking, remove from heat. You can (carefully) peel immediately while running cold water over the hot eggs or you can leave them encased in their shells and peel before eating.

4. In 3 separate meal containers, place 2 eggs, bunch of asparagus, 2–3 ounces salmon, 1–2 slices cheese, and a handful of nuts each, and refrigerate.

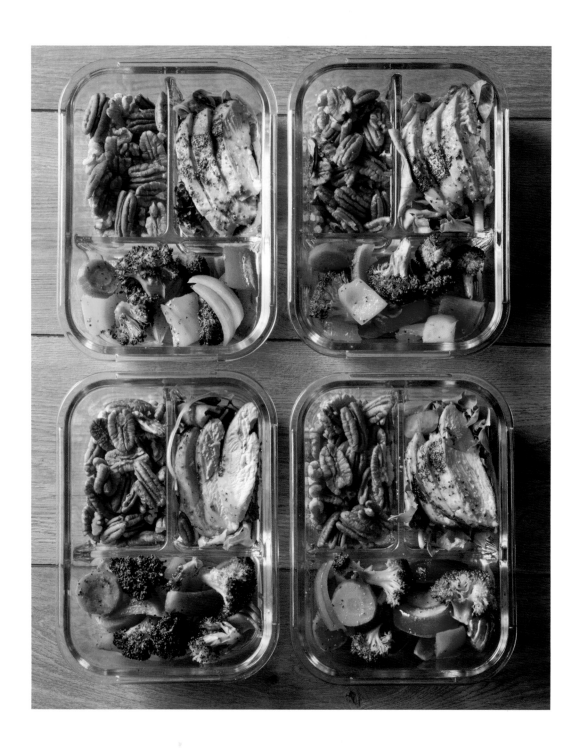

Roasted Chicken and Veggie Lunch Boxes

Serves 1 for 3 days

Ingredients:

1 package broccoli florets
1 red onion, sliced
1 bell pepper, sliced
Oil
Seasonings
1½ pounds chicken breast
3 ounces almonds, pecans,
   or pistachios

Steps:

1. Preheat oven to 350°F.

2. Place broccoli florets and onion and bell pepper slices on a baking sheet.

3. Evenly toss with oil and your favorite seasonings. Make sure everything is in one single layer with little overlapping and roast until tender, around 30 minutes.

4. Meanwhile, grill or pan cook the chicken, using oil and your favorite seasonings.

5. Evenly divide and place the chicken, roasted vegetables, and nuts into 3 separate food containers and refrigerate.

Dinner Option 1:
Cheeseburger with Brussels Sprouts and Cauli Mash

Serves 1 for 2 dinners

Ingredients:

½ small head cauliflower
5-7 whole brussels sprouts
Oil
Seasonings
½ pound ground beef
2–3 tablespoons grated
    Parmesan cheese
1 slice cheese

Steps:

1. Preheat oven to 375°F.

2. Chop cauliflower head into florets and boil or steam using a double boiler until very tender, around 25 minutes. (This vegetable will be used for two dinners, so you can steam the whole head and package half or steam half for each dinner.)

3. While the cauliflower is steaming, slice brussels sprouts in half and toss with oil and favorite seasonings. Place on a baking sheet or dish in a single layer and put in the oven. Roast until tender, around 20 minutes.

4. While the cauliflower is steaming and the brussels sprouts are roasting, form the ground beef into a round patty and add favorite seasonings.

5. Pan cook or grill the burger on one side for 3 minutes; flip over and cook for an additional 4 minutes.

6. While the burger is cooking, place the softened cauliflower in a medium bowl and mash with a fork. Add 2 to 3 tablespoons of grated Parmesan cheese and thoroughly combine until they have a mashed-potato-type texture.

7. Place the slice of cheese on the burger and cook for 1 to 2 more minutes.

8. Plate the burger, mashed cauliflower, and roasted brussels sprouts and serve warm.

Dinner Option 2:
Salmon with Parmesan Roasted Zucchini

Serves 1 for 1 dinner

Ingredients:

1 small zucchini, sliced
Oil
Seasonings
1 salmon fillet
1–2 tablespoons grated
  or shredded Parmesan
  cheese

Steps:

1. Preheat oven to 350°F.

2. Slice the zucchini in long ½-inch-thick strips. Toss with oil until evenly coated and season with your favorite seasonings.

3. Place in the oven and roast until tender, around 15 minutes.

4. Meanwhile, coat both sides of the salmon with oil and season. Grill or pan cook over medium-high heat, skin-side up, for 4 minutes. Flip over and continue to cook until it feels firm, around 3 more minutes or the salmon reaches an internal temperature of 145°F.

5. Sprinkle the tender zucchini with Parmesan cheese and return to the oven for 2 minutes.

6. Plate the salmon and zucchini; serve warm.

Breakfast, Lunch, Dinner Optional Additions

Avocado oil mayo

Butter

Chives

Cilantro

Freshly squeezed lemon

Grated Parmesan cheese

Hot sauce

Lettuce/tomato/onion

Mustard

Oil

Olives

Regular mayo

Seasonings

Shredded cheese

Sliced avocado

Sour cream

Vinegar

Okay! After your first week or so of your 30-day keto plan, you may be ready for something new. Sometimes sticking to some of the same foods (and ones that are devoid of sugar) can seem boring, however, this sometimes comes along with the territory of getting healthy and kicking a sugar habit, so it will all be worth it. Plus, you'll get more comfortable with the recipes and learn to get creative with spices and seasonings! In the next chapter, we will be introducing you to what is commonly known as the "game changer" in the keto community, and that is the "chaffle." Stay tuned!

Chapter 8

Your Keto Solution to Bread, Pizza Dough, Pancakes, and Waffles

If you're like millions of others, not having bread could cause you to completely derail from your 30-day keto plan. We have some delicious solutions for you, and keto dieters swear by them! In this chapter you'll learn about keto-approved bread, pizza dough, pancakes, and waffles (aka "chaffles"). These "bread" products are allowed on the 30-day keto plan because they are uniquely crafted to have the taste and texture of their wheat-based counterparts, however they are made with keto-approved ingredients such as almond flour, coconut flour, cream cheese, and eggs. You will find these ingredients throughout this chapter, however, there are different processes to achieve each outcome.

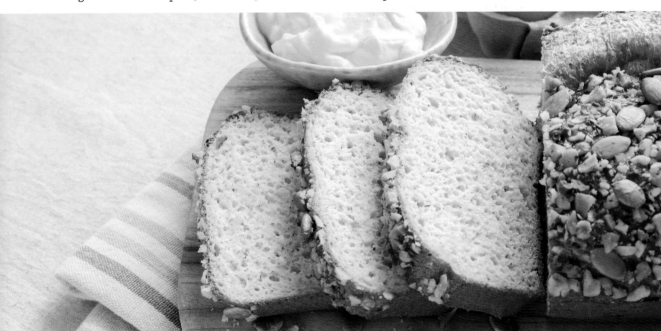

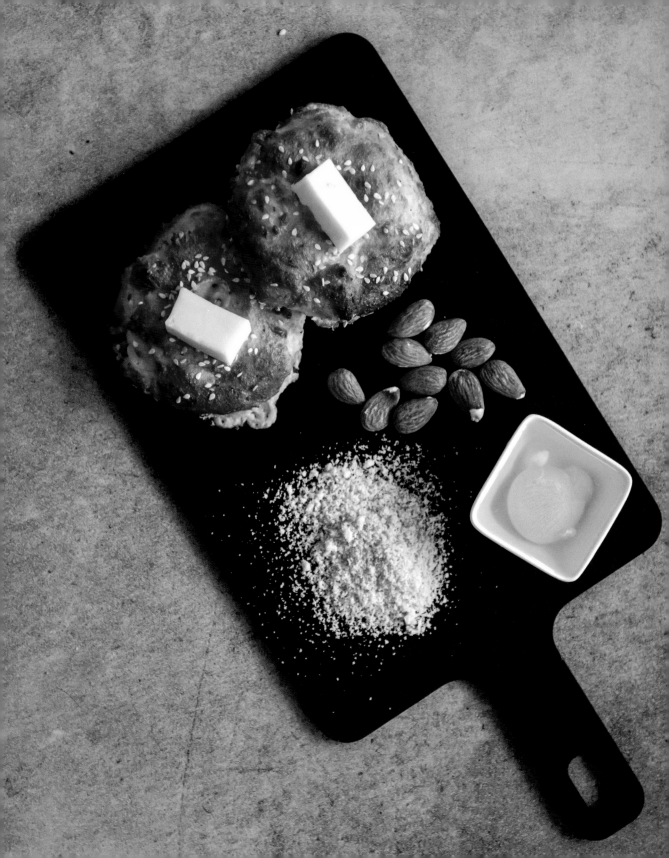

Keto Bread

The term "fathead" bread is well-known and loved in the keto community. It refers to lower-carbohydrate and higher-fat breads that incorporate nut- and coconut-based flours as opposed to wheat flours. The term "fathead" comes from a 2009 documentary where high levels of fat and low levels of carbohydrates were consumed for the leading subject to lose weight. During the film, various doctors and dietitians interviewed stated that based on the latest research in cardiovascular health, it is actually inflammation (as opposed to a diet high in saturated fat) that causes heart disease and heart attacks, some of whom say the inflammation is caused by a high-sugar, high-carbohydrate diet. This "fathead" bread dough is perfect for keto sandwiches, and can be made ahead of time and stored in the refrigerator before baking.

Makes 4 Sandwich Rolls

Ingredients:

¾ cup shredded mozzarella cheese

2 ounces cream cheese

1 egg

⅓ cup almond flour

2 teaspoons baking powder

¼ teaspoon garlic powder

½ cup shredded cheddar cheese

Steps:

1. Place the mozzarella and cream cheese in a microwave-safe bowl. Microwave for 20 seconds at a time on high, until melted.

2. In a medium bowl, whisk the egg. Add the almond flour, baking powder, and garlic powder and combine.

3. Work the mozzarella mixture in with the almond flour mixture until sticky. Stir in the cheddar cheese.

4. Transfer the dough to a sheet of plastic wrap and fold plastic wrap over the dough. Gently work the dough into a ball. Refrigerate for 30 minutes.

5. Preheat the oven to 425°F and grease a baking sheet or line it with parchment paper.

6. Remove dough from refrigerator and unwrap. Cut dough into 4 equal pieces and roll each piece into a ball.

7. Cut each ball in half to form a top and bottom bun. Place the dough, cut sides down, on the prepared baking sheet.

8. Bake until golden, around 10 to 12 minutes.

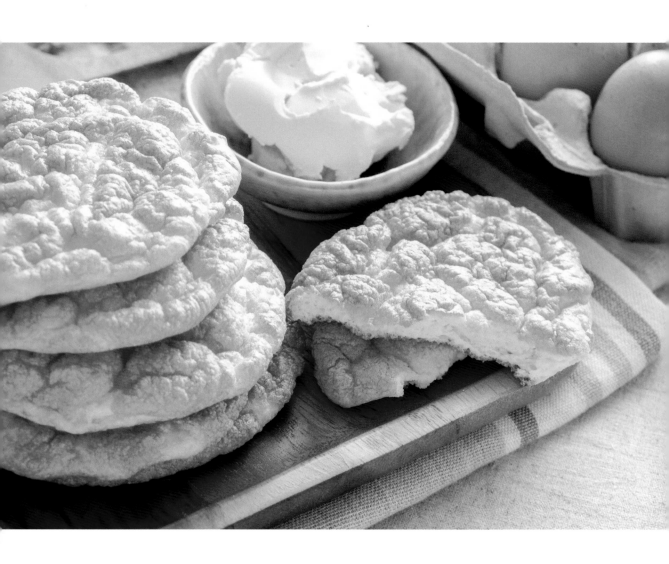

Keto Cloud Bread

Keto cloud bread is another version of a low-carbohydrate bread but it is far more light and airy. It doesn't have too much flavor on its own, so it's the perfect replacement for biscuits with butter or cheese, or for sandwich bread. Another bonus is you only need three ingredients, as this bread does not call for any type of flour alternatives.

Makes 6 Pieces

Ingredients:

Butter or ghee for greasing

3 large eggs, yolks and whites separated

⅛ teaspoon cream of tartar (optional)

3 ounces mascarpone or cream cheese, softened

⅛ teaspoon salt

Steps:

1. Preheat the oven to 300°F. Line a baking sheet with parchment paper and grease lightly with butter or ghee.

2. In large bowl, beat the egg whites and cream of tartar with an electric mixer until you have stiff peaks.

3. In a different large bowl, use the electric mixer to beat the egg yolks, macarpone or cream cheese, and salt until smooth.

4. Gradually (and carefully) fold the egg whites into the cheese mixture with a spatula. Try not to break down the air bubbles of the egg whites.

5. Scoop the mixture into six circular discs on the parchment paper and bake until golden, around 28 to 32 minutes.

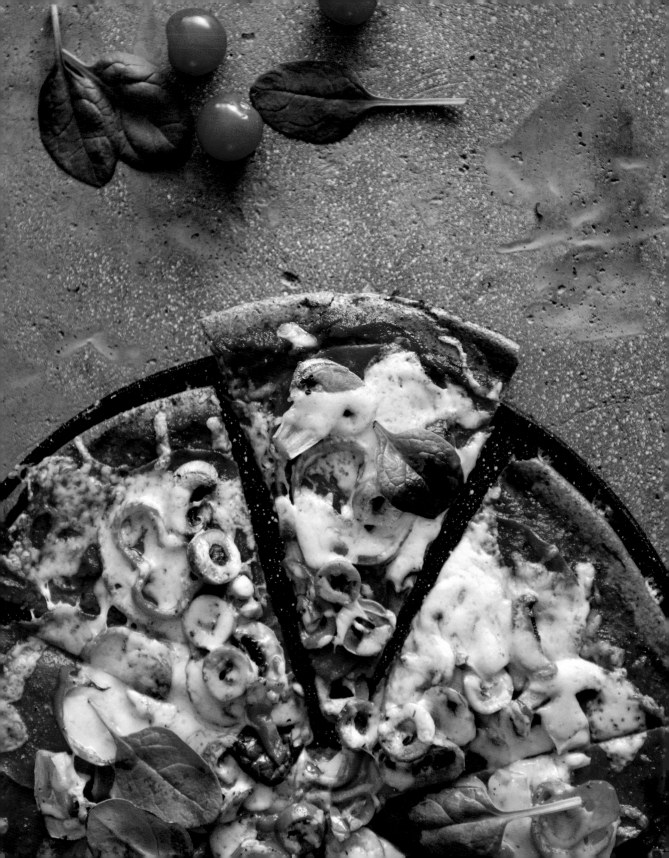

Keto Pizza Dough

Like with keto bread, you may hear keto pizza referred to as "fathead" pizza, and yes, it's the same thing! As with any pizza crust, the process is very important to get the dough just right. The biggest pointer is to keep kneading your dough until it is thoroughly combined and uniform. Also, if it's sticking to your hands, either chill the dough for 20 minutes to make it more manageable, and/or put some oil on your hands to make kneading easier. Feel free to use any keto-approved toppings on your pizza—cheese, sausage, pepperoni, bell peppers, and mushrooms are typical. For a low-sugar pizza sauce, refer to page 263!

Makes 1 Pizza Crust (8 slices)

Ingredients:

1½ cups shredded mozzarella

2 tablespoons cream cheese, cubed

2 large eggs, beaten

⅓ cup coconut flour

Steps:

1. Preheat the oven to 425°F. Line a baking sheet or pizza pan with parchment paper.

2. Combine the shredded mozzarella and cubed cream cheese in a large microwave-safe bowl. Heat for 90 seconds on high, stirring halfway through. Stir again at the end until completely incorporated.

3. Stir in the beaten eggs and coconut flour. Knead with your hands until a dough forms. If the dough hardens before fully combined, microwave for 10 to 15 seconds to soften.

4. Spread the dough onto the lined baking pan to ¼- or ⅓-inch thickness, using your hands or a rolling pin over a piece of parchment paper to prevent the dough from sticking (the rolling pin and parchment paper method works best).

5. Use a toothpick or fork to poke lots of holes throughout the crust to prevent bubbling.

6. Spread low-sugar pizza sauce on top of the crust, followed by cheese, and toppings of choice.

7. Bake for 6 minutes. Poke more holes in any places where you see bubbles forming. Bake for 3 to 7 more minutes, until the edges are golden brown.

Keto Pancake

The keto pancake has almost the same ingredients as found in some of the waffles in the following "chaffle" section. However, if you do not have a waffle griddle, this recipe can be used for a pan. We don't condone the use of syrups with artificial sweeteners during your 30-day keto plan, but you can make a sweet pancake with heavy whipping cream and strawberries. You can also pair this pancake with a fried egg and mashed avocado for a savory breakfast dish.

Makes 1 Large Pancake

Ingredients:

3 tablespoons almond flour
1 large egg
1 teaspoon baking powder
Splash of almond milk
Butter or ghee for cooking

Steps:

1. Using a whisk, thoroughly combine all ingredients.

2. Heat a pan over medium-high heat and melt butter or ghee in the pan.

3. Pour the pancake mixture in the hot pan and wait until you see little holes in the batter as you would with regular pancake batter, around 2 minutes.

4. Flip the pancake over, cook for 1 minute, and serve.

The Chaffle

The chaffle is made with a mini waffle griddle so it looks just like a waffle and has a similar taste and texture. Many (but not all) chaffles are made using cheese, hence the name "chaffle." The original chaffle appeared online not too long ago and it only has two ingredients: ½ cup cheese and 1 egg. Many love this version so we urge you to try it, but some argue this version is too "eggy" and doesn't have the bread texture they are looking for. This chapter provides several chaffle recipes that incorporate more ingredients to achieve the best bread-type texture.

Like we have mentioned previously, we don't endorse the use of artificial sweeteners or even natural zero-calorie sweeteners as it's imperative to get out of the habit of sweetening foods to kick the sugar habit. Due to this we don't use the chaffle for sweet purposes but rather for savory bread replacements—here are some of the most delicious uses.

Bagel
Breakfast sandwiches
Burger bun
Grilled panini sandwich
Pizza
Sandwich bread
Standard waffle
Taco shells

What You Need to Make Chaffles

The good news is you only need one piece of equipment and that's a mini waffle maker. Some make one mini chaffle at a time and some have two griddles which can come in handy. This just depends on how much you want to spend—the single waffle maker is around ten dollars and the double waffle maker is around twenty dollars at most major stores.

The beauty of the chaffle is that the possibilities are endless. You can get creative and use your favorite ingredients to not only make the chaffle itself but also to form a new keto meal with it. Simply combine all of the ingredients and use a nonstick cooking spray (we recommend keto-approved oil sprays as the best choices) to make one chaffle with your mini waffle maker.

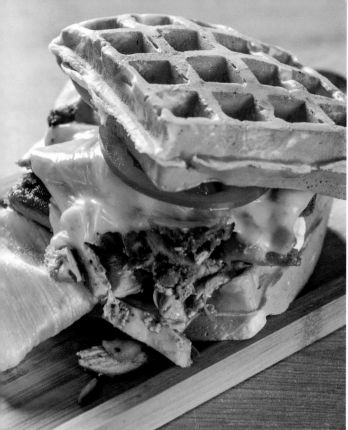

Classic White Bread Chaffle

So many keto dieters agree that this tastes just like white bread so you can use it as sandwich bread, a burger bun, or a grilled panini. Try it stuffed with pulled pork or beef, hamburger, or as a breakfast sandwich with egg, cheese, and bacon.

Ingredients:

3 tablespoons almond flour

¼ teaspoon baking powder

1 teaspoon water

1 egg

1 tablespoon mayonnaise

The Nut-Free Chaffle

This chaffle is the nut-free counterpart of the classic white bread chaffle found above. It will have the same taste but it's actually a little bit fluffier!

Ingredients:

1 tablespoon coconut flour

1 tablespoon water

1 tablespoon mayonnaise

⅛ teaspoon baking powder

1 egg

⅛ teaspoon salt

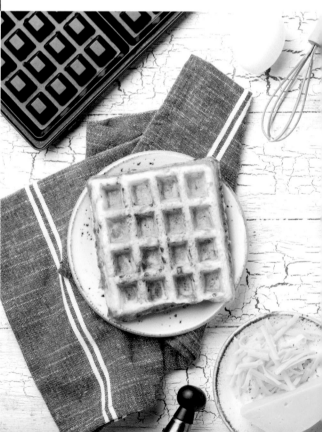

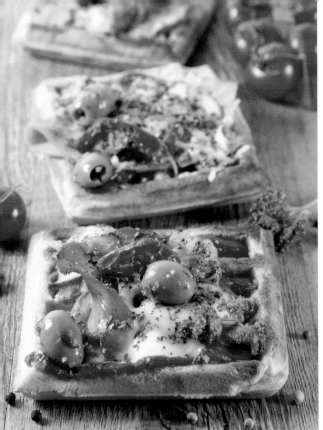

Pizza Chaffle

The pizza chaffle can be eaten on its own or you can top with more of your favorite pizza toppings such as extra cheese, tomatoes, olives, and prosciutto.

Ingredients:

1 egg
¼ cup Italian cheese blend
1 tablespoon sugar-free pizza sauce
2 tablespoons pepperoni, diced

Lox Bagel Chaffle

If you love a bagel with cream cheese and lox, this is your chaffle! If you aren't near a Trader Joe's grocery store, which sells its famous "Everything but the Bagel" seasoning, simply replace with a few dashes of sesame seeds, garlic powder, dried minced onion, and salt to taste. After making your chaffles, simply top with cream cheese and smoked salmon—other optional additions are sliced cucumber and/or radish.

Ingredients:

1 egg
¼ cup mozzarella cheese
1 tablespoon cream cheese
2 tablespoons almond flour
¼ teaspoon baking powder
Everything but the Bagel seasoning, to taste

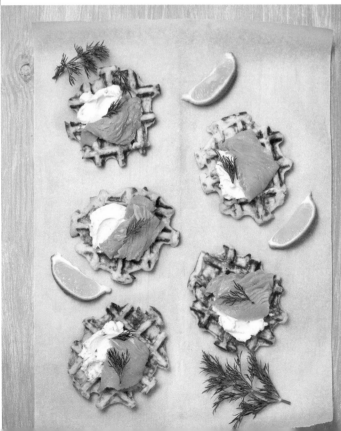

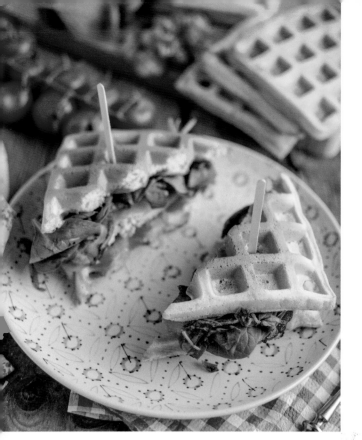

Stuffing Chaffle

If you like leftover holiday turkey sandwiches, you'll love the stuffing chaffle. Many elements of classic turkey stuffing are in this chaffle, so this is the perfect "bread" for a turkey sandwich.

Ingredients:

3 tablespoons almond flour

¼ teaspoon baking powder

1 teaspoon water

1 egg

1 tablespoon mayonnaise

1 diced celery stalk + 1 tablespoon diced onion, sautéed

Poultry seasoning, sage, and thyme, to taste

Cheddar Chaffle

This chaffle has cheesy flavor, so it is great for any sandwich where cheese may make a nice addition. Chicken salad and tuna salad sandwiches, bacon lettuce tomato (BLT), or standard ham and tomato sandwiches are popular ways to use this chaffle.

Ingredients:

1 egg

½ cup shredded cheddar cheese

1 teaspoon garlic salt

2 tablespoons almond flour

½ teaspoon baking powder

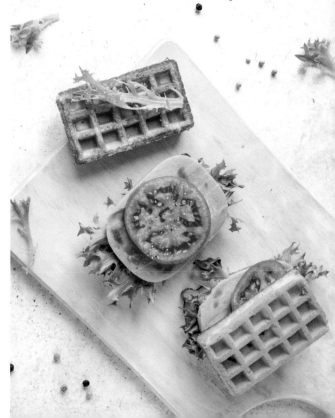

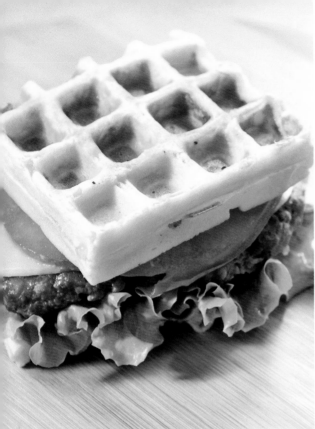

Mozzarella Chaffle

This chaffle is the mozzarella version of the cheddar chaffle and can be used in the same manner. It goes well with sandwiches and burgers especially when mozzarella cheese is one of the additions.

Ingredients:

1 egg
½ cup shredded mozzarella cheese
1 teaspoon garlic salt
2 tablespoons almond flour
½ teaspoon baking powder

Standard Breakfast Chaffle

This recipe is the closest one to a traditional breakfast waffle if you were to add syrup and butter. Since the 30-day keto plan doesn't use added sweeteners, you can make a savory pairing with eggs and mashed avocado.

Ingredients:

2 eggs
2 tablespoons cream cheese
2 tablespoons almond flour
1 tablespoon coconut oil or melted butter
½ teaspoon baking powder

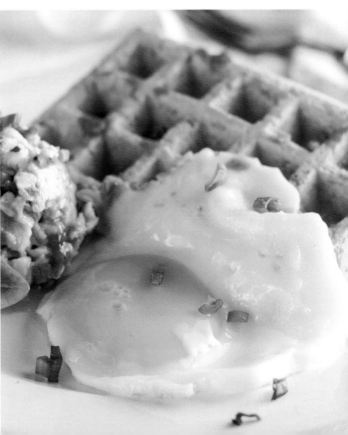

Batch Cooking the Chaffle

In the coming chapter about batch cooking, you will learn how to make several meals in one cooking session that can be stored in the refrigerator or freezer. You can implement this strategy with chaffles as well, since they keep well in the refrigerator and freezer, and can simply be reheated by using your toaster. They may not be quite as crispy as the freshly made chaffles, but they come out pretty close!

We hope this chapter provides some variety in your nutrition plan with a keto-approved food that can double as bread, burger buns, bagels, and more. If you're like thousands of other keto dieters and love the chaffle, you can use it as a staple food and construct your meal plan around it. The recipes found in this chapter can be used for many simple ideas, however, the possibilities are endless, so feel free to use your favorite (low-carb and low-sugar) ingredients to make your favorite chaffle.

Chapter 9

Restaurant Keto

I f you have absolutely no time for food prepping, or you just have zero interest or motivation to pack food for work, you can still complete the 30-day keto plan. In today's society, it's commonplace to grab food (even every day!) during your lunch hour in a restaurant or takeout establishment. This is reality for many of us, so we want to provide a strategy for keto weight loss even if you're a frequent restaurant goer. Let's face it, life happens (and so do work luncheons, birthdays, and other social gatherings), and we want you to have options so you can live your life accordingly for the month. Many think they have to give up their social lives or drastically rearrange their eating schedule at the office to adhere to a 30-day plan, and that can lead to procrastination for even starting a nutrition plan due to strict limitations. Yes, you can still go to restaurants and enjoy wonderful company (and maybe even a glass of wine . . . or two).

As we have mentioned previously, fast food is not allowed on the 30-day keto plan because we want you to achieve wellness in addition to weight loss. We have heard countless stories of keto dieters sticking to the proper macronutrients of fats, carbohydrates, and proteins by frequenting the fast-food drive-through and ordering a bunless double (or triple) cheeseburger with mayonnaise, along with a diet soda. It's an easy habit to get into since it's convenient, relatively cheap, and pretty tasty! Especially if you're new to keto and learning the ropes, we want to set the healthiest foundation possible and instruct readers how to get the best nutrition from this type of food plan since choosing detrimental foods (even while hitting your macronutrient requirements) can lead to unfavorable outcomes. Many people have reported adverse effects such as drastically increased bad cholesterol, sodium, and even hospitalization when following a "dirty keto" nutrition plan which consists of a large percentage of fast food, deli meats, inferior oils, and processed foods.

Dining establishments that are included on the 30-day plan are:

- National chain dine-in restaurants
- Smaller boutique dine-in restaurants
- Takeout restaurants that offer salads, sandwiches (lettuce-wrapped), and platters with choices of unprocessed meats and vegetables
- Coffee shops

You'll want to avoid:

- Standard fast-food establishments
- Almost anything with a drive-through
- Pizza parlors
- Takeout places that only offer processed deli meats

It's convenient to look online at restaurant menus before choosing where to grab your meal as some have far more keto-approved options than others. If you end up somewhere without looking at food options first, not to worry—you can get a keto meal almost anywhere nowadays! Of course you may have to modify your order, but making simple substitutions will turn a high-glycemic meal into a keto-friendly one quite easily. Here are nine common restaurant scenarios that typically include high-carbohydrate and high-sugar foods, as well as keto-friendly replacement options.

Scenario One: You're at a typical café, and the server arrives with a basket of bread and butter.

Solution 1: Before the bread even touches the table, just say "no thanks!"—you'll be eating a full meal soon anyway.

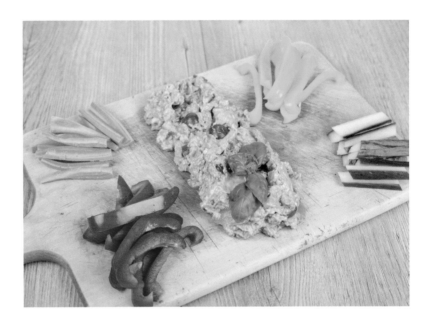

Solution 2: Replace with a high-fat dip and veggies.

Solution 3: Replace with a cream-based soup, but check with the server about the exact ingredients to make sure there are no grain-based fillers or thickeners.

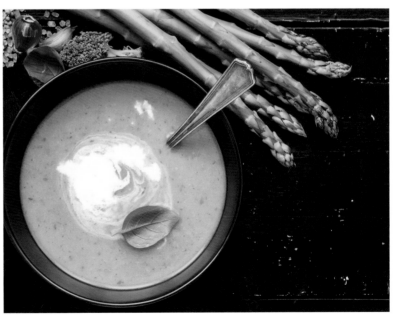

Scenario Two: You're at a more casual takeout place with sandwiches, salads, and burgers.

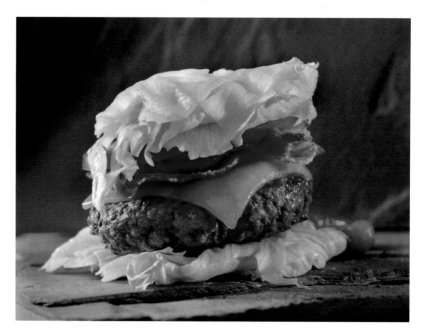

Solution 1: Just get it lettuce wrapped—most restaurants will oblige. Sorry, no fries, but a side of green vegetables will do!

Solution 2: A hearty salad with protein and fats that will keep you satiated—choose a dressing that is typically low in sugar such as oil and vinegar or Caesar.

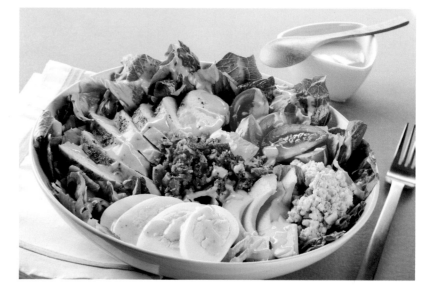

Scenario Three: You're at an Italian eatery and everyone is getting pizza and those types of flavors sound really appetizing.

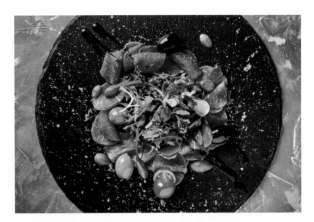

Solution 1: Beef carpaccio with additions such as arugula, cheese, olives, and tomatoes.

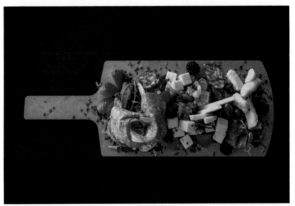

Solution 2: If you haven't had too many servings of processed meats recently, a meat and cheese charcuterie board.

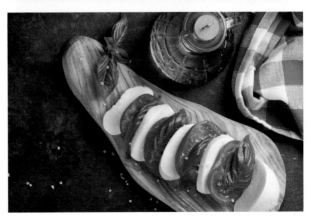

Solution 3: Caprese salad topped with olive oil.

Scenario Four: You're at a typical chain restaurant with standard meals that contain a protein with side dishes of pasta, rice, and potatoes.

Solution 1: Ask your server to remove all high-carbohydrate side dishes and replace with low-carbohydrate produce.

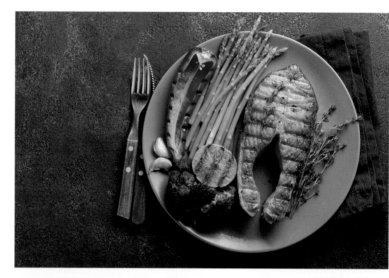

Solution 2: Ask your server to remove all high-carbohydrate sides dishes and ask to replace with one green vegetable with a cheese, cream, or butter-based sauce.

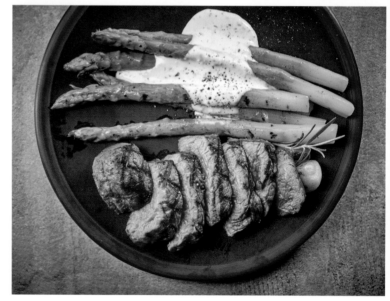

Scenario Five: You're at happy hour with friends for drinks and small plates.

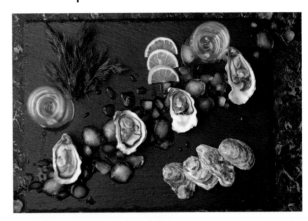

Solution 1: You celebrate your new keto lifestyle with brut sparkling wine and oysters.

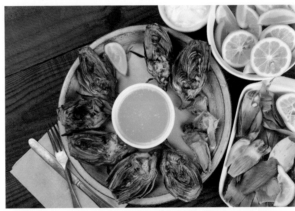

Solution 2: You pair a buttery chardonnay with a steamed artichoke with mayo and butter for dipping.

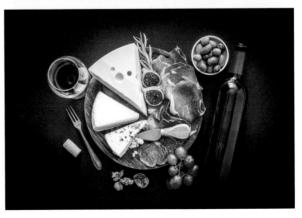

Solution 3: You relax with a glass of cabernet sauvignon and cheese board with nuts and olives.

Scenario Six: You're grabbing Mexican food for Taco Tuesday.

Solution 1: Shrimp, steak, or chicken fajitas with guacamole, shredded cheese, and salsa—ask for lettuce cups or eat as a platter.

Solution 2: Chile verde platter of pork, green sauce, sour cream, and guacamole—skip the rice, beans, and tortillas!

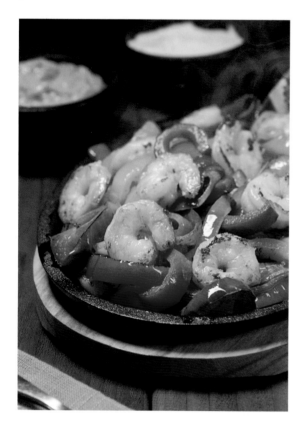
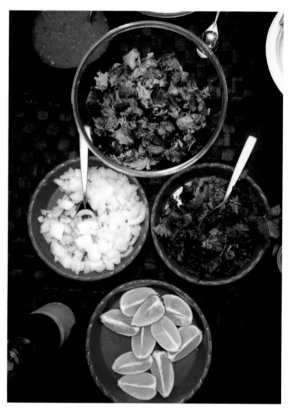

Scenario Seven: You're out for Chinese or Vietnamese food, or for sushi.

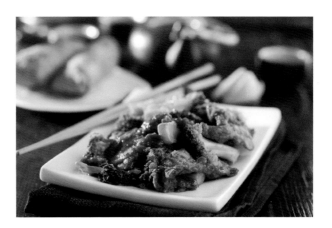

Solution 1: Beef and broccoli and egg drop soup instead of a noodle dish.

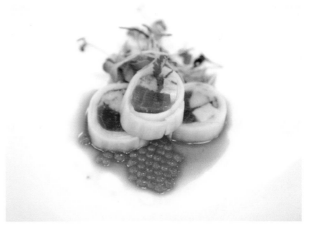

Solution 2: At sushi, instead of a roll with rice, ask for it to be wrapped in cucumber—this, too, is a standard option on most menus (look for a Naruto roll)!

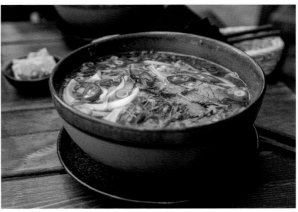

Solution 3: Vietnamese pho (meat, noodle, herb, and vegetable soup)—ask for no noodles and extra veggies and herbs—this is a standard option on most menus!

Scenario Eight: You pop into Starbucks before work.

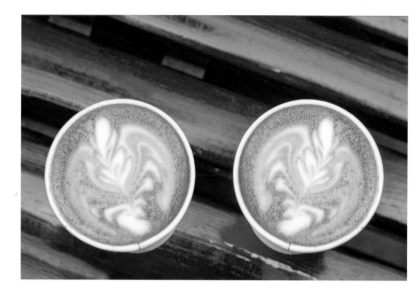

Solution 1: A grande coffee with heavy cream or almond milk, or a grande latte made with heavy cream instead of milk.

Solution 2: Egg bites (eggs with cheese and veggies, or eggs with cheese and bacon), string cheese, and mashed avocado. These items are offered à la carte and make an easy keto-approved breakfast on the go.

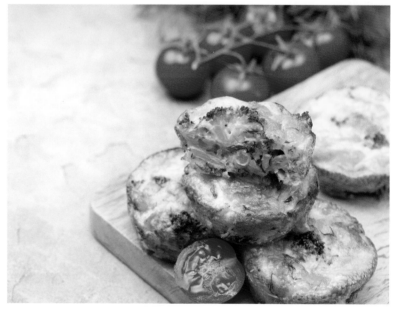

Scenario Nine: You're out to breakfast or brunch with family and friends.

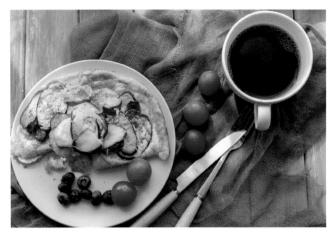

Solution 1: Omelet with vegetables, cheese, and sausage with small side of tomatoes and/or berries, and coffee.

Solution 2: Eggs Benedict with no bread base (most restaurants will make it this way); ask to add fresh produce such as asparagus, tomatoes, and mushrooms.

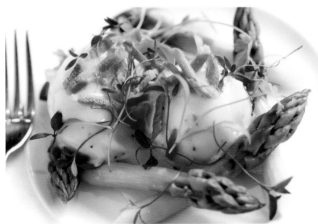

Contrary to popular belief, the keto nutrition plan can be achieved even if you frequent restaurants—you just have to be meticulous about your order! Of course, we do advise to try to limit your restaurant outings during your 30-day keto plan, since restaurants may use inferior oils, lots of salt, and possible hidden ingredients. If that's just not realistic for you given your lifestyle, you can still get the weight-loss results by following the simple guidelines found in this chapter.

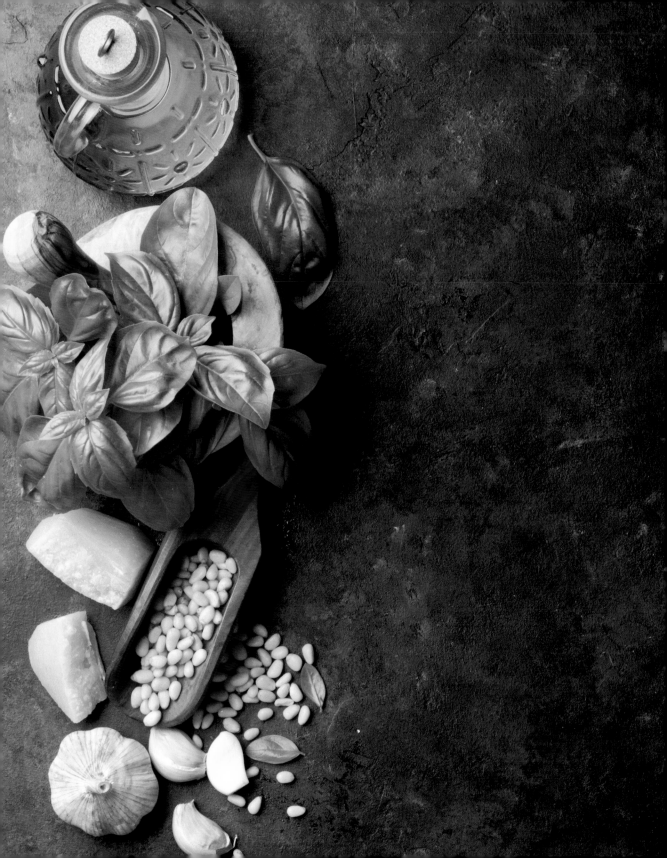

Chapter 10

Advanced Batch Cooking

Wouldn't it be nice if healthy meals were delivered or (even better) if you had a personal chef to whip up dinner for you each night after a long day of work? Or maybe even one of those pricey food-delivery services could take the stress out of cooking every single night. Not having these atypical luxuries makes sticking to a regimented food plan quite difficult sometimes as laboring away in the kitchen between work and family can be impossible at times.

There is a process that several people employ to help get as close as possible to having ready-made healthy meals each evening (or even each morning and afternoon) without hiring a meal service or personal chef, and this technique is called batch cooking. Reflecting its name, batch cooking means exactly that—preparing and cooking large portions of meals all at once so you can keep extra in the freezer or fridge to simply unfreeze and/or reheat future meals. If you have never batch-cooked before, it's easier than you may think, which quickly became apparent to so many people during the Covid-19 quarantine, when an extreme amount of people suddenly found themselves not only with extra time on their hands to learn and experiment, but also a majority of restaurants temporarily closed. When everyone is back to regular hectic schedules, your newly found talent of batch cooking will come in very handy!

Besides the fact that batch cooking helps you to stay prepared and on track with your goals, it also cuts down on food waste. Astonishingly, the average American throws away 219 *pounds* of food every year.[1] When you batch cook, you can prepare several different recipes that use the same ingredients, so you never have to find that flimsy, wilted half

---

1   "Food Waste in America in 2020: Statistics & Facts: RTS," accessed June 10, 2020, rts.com/resources/guides/food-waste -america/.

head of broccoli in the back of your refrigerator ever again. The process allows you to create an abundance of premade meals before your groceries expire and go to waste.

The 219 pounds of wasted food I previously mentioned can equate to upward of $800 also in the trash, meaning batch cooking will save you money. In addition to the money saved in groceries that are consumed as opposed to thrown away, when you know you have already prepared meals at home, temptation to swing by the drive-through or succumb to a bag of potato chips after walking in the door from work will be mitigated. The two-pronged benefit of saving money and sticking to your health goals makes batch cooking a worthwhile skill to have.

The easiest way to start is by making larger portions—simply double or triple the dinner you were already planning. Since you'll already have the cutting boards, knives, pots, and pans out (and you'll have to clean up those items), and you'll be preparing and cooking a dinner for two, you may as well make more food that can be refrigerated and eaten later that week. Essentially, you'll produce six meals in almost the same amount of time that it would take to produce two.

Even if you don't want to dedicate a whole Sunday afternoon to preparing, cooking, and freezing ten or even twenty meals (like some do), all you have to do is triple your dinner recipe a few times per week and you'll definitely start to build up a stash! For example, if you're making your favorite casserole, simply make more and portion it into freezer bags. A simple reheat from the microwave will give you another hot meal when you're too busy to cook. This moderate and gradual way to batch cook is my favorite as it doesn't seem to make much more effort than cooking a standard dinner—no saying goodbye to Sunday afternoons!

Using crossover ingredients is another key to batch cooking. There are some foods that are common in a variety of meals—let's take onions, for example. Onions are found in casseroles, soups, stir-fries, and more, and how many times have you found that shriveled up half onion in the back of your produce drawer? If you're going to slice one quarter of an onion for one meal, you may as well just slice the whole thing or even two whole onions to create a number of meals.

For us, the biggest crossover foods are proteins—you can use them in so many different dishes and they are usually the most time consuming to prepare so having an already cooked batch of meat, chicken, or fish in the fridge is very convenient. It's common for me to cook and store up to two pounds of chicken breast at one time—I'll have enough chicken to last me through the week. I use it to add to salads or lettuce wrapped tacos, and even just on its own to dip in avocado oil mayo or guacamole.

If you're like us and only like to batch cook enough meals for a few days, you won't need a freezer but if you become a batch-cooking pro, you will need to become very familiar with how to freeze foods properly. Knowing what you can and can't freeze is step one, and you will find after a quick Google search that most foods (except things like lettuce and cream cheese) can be frozen and reheated. Knowing how long you can freeze for is step two—meat, seafood, soups, stews, and casseroles can be frozen for up to three months while vegetables can be frozen for up to eight months. Finally, make sure to freeze in the actual portions you will be eating and label everything by name and date frozen.

In chapter 7, we provided smaller batch-cooking ideas for breakfast and lunch for two to three days, however, this chapter focuses on meal planning for a full workweek, using the batch-cooking method for lunches and dinners. Typically, making a simple keto breakfast, one day at a time, either right before work or the night before doesn't take much time at all as long as you stick to easy expedited breakfast ideas. Of course they won't be overly fancy dishes, but we are focusing on achieving results and sticking to the 30-day plan as easily, efficiently, and inexpensively as possible. This batch-cooking example plan provides recipes for delicious lunches and dinners that can be refrigerated for the standard five-day workweek and the denoted freezer-friendly meals can be frozen for much longer (simply multiply the recipe by two if you would like ten meals, by three if you would like fifteen meals, and so on).

Instructions: The batch-cooking plan below (and recipes to follow) can potentially fulfill your entire 30-day keto nutrition plan, however, many like to batch cook for the work-week and then have more flexibility on the weekends. If you prefer to eat different foods (or even go to restaurants) on the weekends, simply choose four Monday-through-Friday batch-cooking plans below and construct your weekend meal plan with other foods and recipes found in this book. Recipes for all meals found in this batch-cooking plan will follow and you will also find two alternate recipes near the end of this chapter for more variety. Go ahead and bookmark or put sticky notes on the recipe pages for your chosen meal plan! Your expedited breakfast can be prepared in ten minutes or less, each morning. If you choose to dine out, the restaurant guidelines found in chapter 9 will provide guidance.

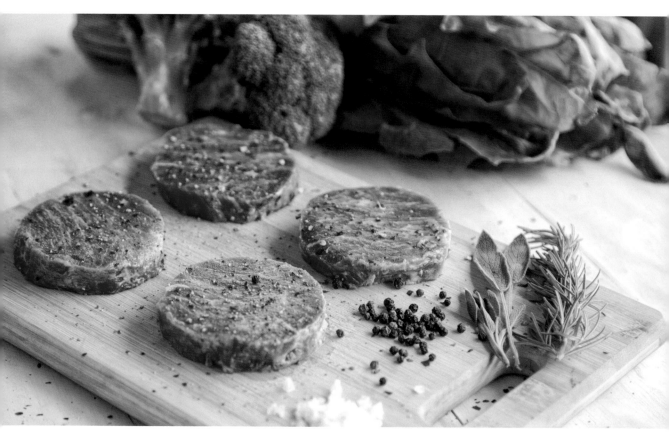

Meals/Days	Breakfast (Pick One)	Lunch	Dinner	Snacks
Monday–Friday Option One	Choose 1 Expedited Breakfast option	Classic chicken salad (batch cook)	Hamburger cauliflower casserole (batch cook)*	Piece of cheese Serving of nuts
Monday–Friday Option Two	Choose 1 Expedited Breakfast option	Turkey chili (batch cook)*	Chicken Alfredo bowls (batch cook)*	Celery sticks with mashed avocado Serving of olives
Monday–Friday Option Three	Choose 1 Expedited Breakfast option	Hearty Broccoli Salad (batch cook)	Bun-less Philly cheese steak platter (batch cook)*	2 squares of dark chocolate Piece of cheese
Monday–Friday Option Four	Choose 1 Expedited Breakfast option	Gyro meatball salad (batch cook)	Cheesy chicken in green sauce (batch cook)*	Coconut cream with raspberries Serving of nuts
Monday–Friday Option Five	Choose 1 Expedited Breakfast option	Mayo-free tuna salad (batch cook)	Chinese pulled pork with mashed cauliflower (batch cook)*	Celery with nut butter Keto coffee
Monday–Friday Option Six	Choose 1 Expedited Breakfast option	Turkey burger with roasted squash and veggies (batch cook)	Creamy cod casserole (batch cook)*	Salami slices with cream cheese Serving of nuts

*These recipes are freezer-friendly.

Expedited Breakfast Ideas

Keto coffee (page 185)

Plain coffee with cream, butter, or ghee

2–3 eggs your way with optional sides of tomatoes, avocado, or berries

Scrambled eggs topped with cheese, avocado, salsa

Plain yogurt (Greek, almond, coconut) topped with berries, nut butter, and hemp seeds

Chia seed pudding (page 187)

Cottage cheese with berries

Breakfast charcuterie box (hard-boiled egg, celery with cream cheese, smoked salmon, nuts, berries)

Gyro Meatball Salad

Meatball Ingredients:

¾ pound ground beef
¾ pound ground lamb
2 large eggs
⅓ cup finely chopped yellow onion
2 tablespoons minced garlic
2 teaspoons ground cumin
1 teaspoon dried oregano
Salt and pepper, to taste
½ cup crumbled feta cheese

Salad Ingredients:

20 cherry tomatoes, halved
1 red bell pepper, thinly sliced
½ red onion, thinly sliced
1 cucumber, thinly sliced
Leafy greens (optional)
1 batch Tzatziki Dipping Sauce (page 265)

Steps:

1. Preheat oven to 400°F and line a baking sheet with parchment paper.

2. In a large bowl, combine all meatball ingredients (except the feta cheese) thoroughly with your hands.

3. Gently fold the feta cheese into the meatball mixture.

4. Form the mixture into 26 1-inch meatballs and place on the lined baking sheet, 1 inch apart.

5. Bake for 20 to 25 minutes, until the outside of the meatballs are browned and the internal temperature reaches 160°F.

6. Meanwhile, combine the tomatoes, bell pepper, red onion, and cucumber in medium bowl and toss. Add in leafy greens (optional).

7. Divide the salad between five airtight containers and refrigerate.

8. After the meatballs have cooled enough to handle, divide into the five containers and refrigerate.

9. To serve, reheat the meatballs or enjoy cold. Scoop desired amount of Tzatziki Dipping Sauce into the salad container to use for dip.

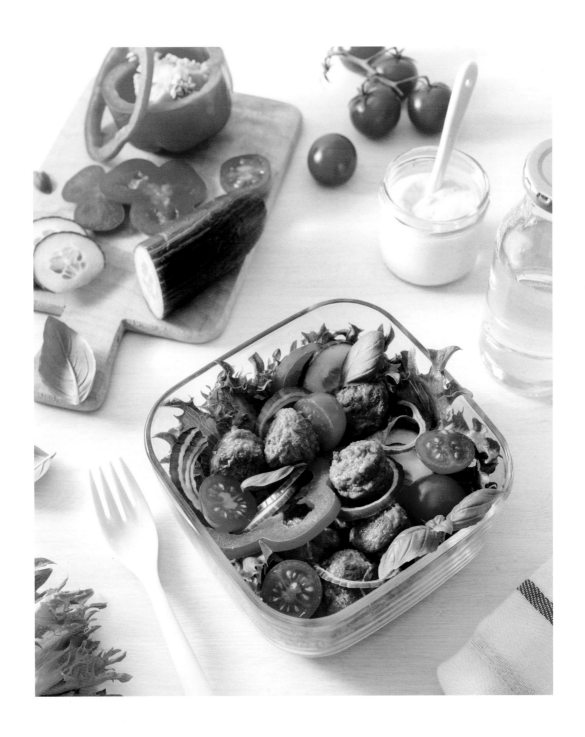

Hearty Broccoli Salad

Salad Ingredients:

3 large heads broccoli, cut into bite-size pieces

¾ cup shredded cheddar cheese

⅓ red onion, thinly sliced

¼ cup sliced almonds

4 slices bacon, cooked and crumbled

3 green onions, chopped

Diced avocado for garnish (optional)

Dressing Ingredients:

⅔ cup mayonnaise

3 tablespoons apple cider vinegar

1 tablespoon Dijon mustard

Salt and pepper, to taste

Steps:

1. In a medium saucepan over high heat, bring 6 cups of water to a boil. In the meantime, prepare a large bowl with ice water.

2. Add the broccoli florets to the boiling water and cook until slightly tender, around 2 to 3 minutes. Remove with a slotted spoon and place in the ice water to stop the cooking process. Once all broccoli has been cooled in the water, strain with a colander and place in a large bowl.

3. In a medium bowl, whisk all dressing ingredients together until combined. Pour the dressing over the broccoli and toss until all broccoli is coated.

4. Add all other salad ingredients to the bowl except for the avocado and toss for 30 seconds, until combined.

5. Divide between five airtight containers and refrigerate. Add diced avocado before serving (optional).

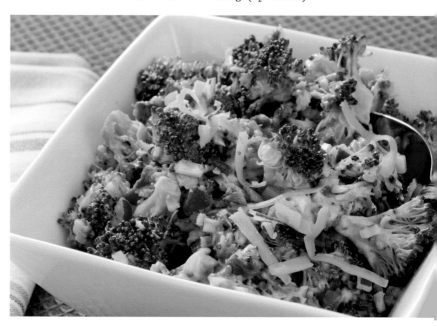

White Turkey Chili

Ingredients:

3 tablespoons coconut oil
1 small onion, diced
3 garlic cloves, minced
1½ pounds ground turkey
    (or beef, lamb, or pork)
Your favorite seasonings,
    to taste
3 cups riced cauliflower
3 cups full-fat coconut milk
2 tablespoons mustard

Steps:

1. In a large pot, heat the coconut oil. Add the onion and garlic. Stir for 2 to 3 minutes and then add the ground turkey.

2. Break up with the spatula and stir constantly until crumbled. Add in your favorite seasonings and riced cauliflower, and stir well.

3. Once the meat is browned add in the coconut milk and mustard, bring to a simmer, and reduce for 5 to 8 minutes, stirring often.

4. Divide between five airtight containers and refrigerate.

5. To serve, reheat and eat on its own or top with shredded cheese, avocado, sour cream, and salsa.

Mayo-free Tuna Salad

Ingredients:

5 cans tuna packed in water
½ red onion, diced
4 celery stalks, diced
⅓ cup fresh dill, chopped
3 tablespoons extra-virgin
    olive oil
1 tablespoon apple cider
    vinegar
1 tablespoon Dijon mustard
Juice from 2 lemons
3 hard-boiled eggs, diced
Salt and pepper, to taste
Celery sticks or endive
    leaves to dip

Steps:

1. Place tuna in large bowl and break up, using a fork. Add in the onion, celery, and dill.

2. In a small bowl, whisk together the oil, vinegar, mustard, and lemon juice. Pour the dressing over the tuna mixture and thoroughly combine so all tuna is covered.

3. Gently fold the diced eggs into the mixture and season with salt and pepper, to taste.

4. Divide between five airtight containers and refrigerate. Serve cold with celery sticks or endive leaves for dippers or on a bed of greens.

Classic Chicken Salad

Ingredients:

1 cooked rotisserie chicken
½ small onion, diced
3 celery stalks, diced
⅔ cup avocado oil
   mayonnaise
⅓ cup pecans, chopped
2 teaspoons apple cider
   vinegar
Salt and pepper, to taste

Steps:

1. Chop or shred the chicken meat, while removing bones.

2. In a large bowl, combine all remaining ingredients with the chicken.

3. Section into 5 small, airtight containers and refrigerate. Serve on its own, with celery stick dippers, or wrapped in lettuce with your favorite veggies.

No-Tortilla Cheesy Chicken Enchiladas in Green Sauce

Ingredients:

2 tablespoons oil
2 pounds chicken breast,
   chopped
12 ounces tomatillo sauce
   (salsa verde)
2 cups Mexican blend
   shredded cheese
Avocado, sour cream,
   cilantro for serving
   (optional)

Steps:

1. In a large pan over medium-high heat, heat the oil and place the chopped chicken in the pan.

2. Cook for 3 minutes and then flip the chicken pieces over with a spatula. Reduce heat to medium.

3. Continue to cook until chicken is almost cooked through, around 8 minutes, while stirring occasionally.

4. Add the tomatillo sauce and simmer for 3 more minutes.

5. Divide into five servings and place into airtight containers. Top the containers with equal amounts of shredded cheese.

6. Reheat to serve and top with avocado, sour cream, and cilantro (optional).

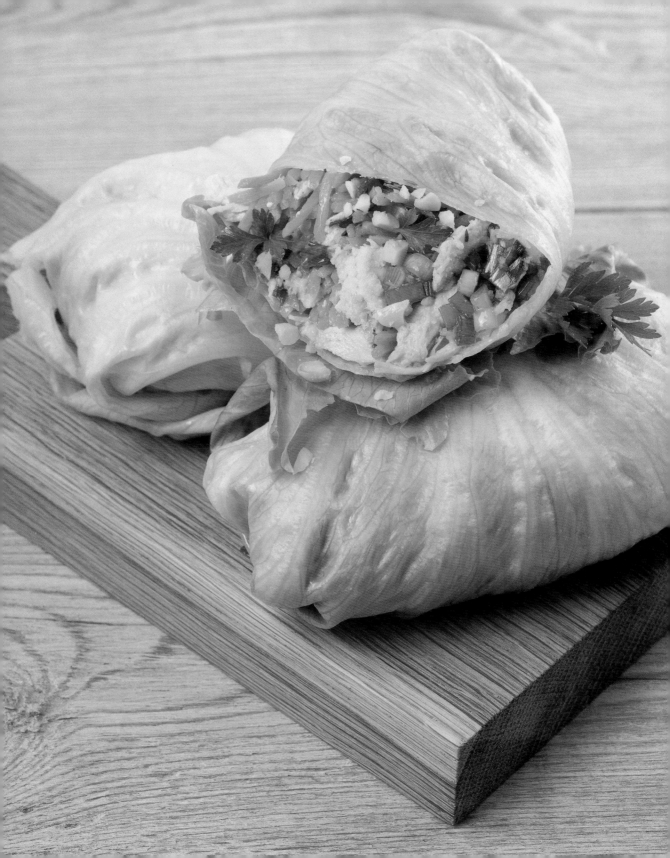

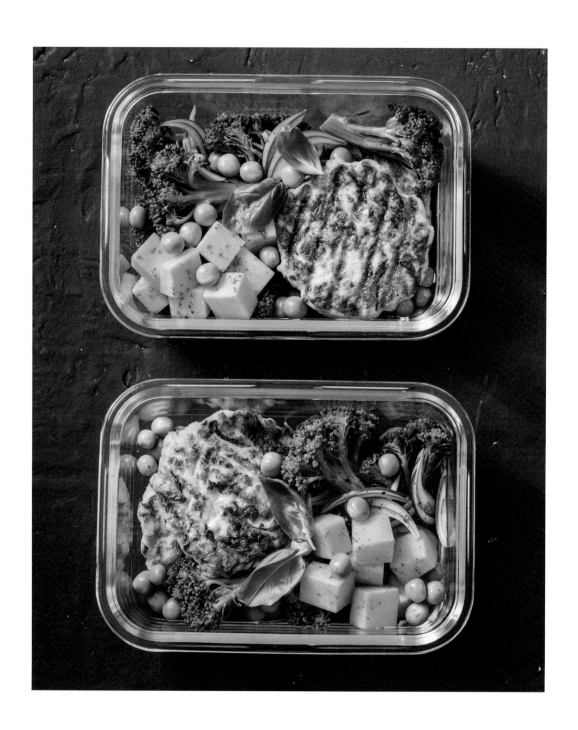

Turkey Burgers with Roasted Squash and Veggies

Ingredients:

4 cups broccoli florets

2 cups cubed butternut squash

½ red onion, sliced

4 tablespoons oil, divided

1 teaspoon dried thyme

Salt and pepper, to taste

2 pounds ground turkey meat

Your favorite seasonings, to taste

Cheese, mayonnaise, mustard, and avocado for serving (optional)

Steps:

1. Preheat oven to 425°F and cover a baking sheet or roasting pan with parchment paper.

2. In a large bowl combine the broccoli, squash, onion, 3 tablespoons of oil, thyme, salt, and pepper. Toss thoroughly to evenly coat.

3. Spread onto the baking sheet and roast for 25 to 30 minutes until the squash is fork tender and the broccoli crisp, tossing them once halfway through.

4. Meanwhile, divide the turkey meat into five patties and season to taste. Using the remaining oil, pan cook over medium-high heat for 3 minutes and browned on one side. Flip over and reduce heat to medium and cook through, around 8 minutes, flipping occasionally.

5. Divide the broccoli and squash mixture between five airtight containers and top each with one turkey burger, and refrigerate.

6. To serve, reheat and top turkey burger with one slice of cheese, and serve with mayonnaise, mustard, and avocado (optional).

Chicken and Broccoli Alfredo Bowls

Ingredients:

2 tablespoons butter

¾ cup yellow onion, diced

2 cloves garlic, minced

8 ounces white mushrooms, sliced

1½ pounds chicken breasts or thighs, cubed and cooked (you can use already prepared rotisserie chicken)

3 cups broccoli florets, steamed

2 cups store-bought or homemade Alfredo sauce (page 262)

Chopped parsley, for garnish (optional)

Steps:

1. Melt the butter in a large skillet over medium heat. Add the onions, garlic, and mushrooms, and cook until the onions are translucent and the mushrooms are cooked through, around 7 minutes.

2. Add the chicken, steamed broccoli, and Alfredo sauce. Combine and simmer for 3 minutes.

3. Divide between five meal storage containers and refrigerate. To serve, reheat and top with chopped parsley (optional).

Bun-less Philly Cheese Steak Platter

Ingredients:

3 tablespoons butter

2 cups white mushrooms, sliced

1 cup chopped onions

1 cup chopped green bell pepper

Garlic powder, to taste

1½ pounds rare roast beef slices

Salt and pepper, to taste

10 slices provolone cheese (for serving)

Steps:

1. In a large saucepan over medium heat, melt the butter. Add the mushrooms, onions, bell peppers, and garlic powder. Cook until the mixture is tender, around 6 to 7 minutes.

2. Cut the roast beef into 1-inch squares and add to the saucepan.

3. Toss with the mushrooms, onions, and bell peppers for 2 minutes until heated through. Add salt and pepper, to taste.

4. Divide between five airtight containers and refrigerate.

5. To serve, reheat and top with two slices provolone cheese.

Hamburger Cauliflower Casserole

Ingredients:

2 small heads cauliflower
1½ pounds ground beef
1 teaspoon cumin
1 teaspoon paprika
1 teaspoon dried oregano
Salt and pepper, to taste
2 large eggs
1½ cups coconut milk or
    heavy whipping cream
1½ cups chicken broth

Steps:

1. Preheat oven to 350°F.

2. Cut the cauliflower into uniform bite-size pieces.

3. Using a steamer pot over high heat, steam the cauliflower until barely tender, around 6 to 7 minutes, and remove from heat and set aside, uncovered.

4. Place the ground beef in a large pan over medium heat and season with cumin, paprika, oregano, salt, and pepper.

5. Break up the ground beef while cooking.

6. In a medium bowl, beat the eggs, cream, and broth until combined. Season with salt and pepper.

7. In a casserole dish, layer the ground beef on the bottom, and then top with an even layer of cooked cauliflower.

8. Pour the egg mixture over the beef and cauliflower, covering it all.

9. Bake until the center is set, around 40 to 45 minutes.

10. Serve warm or divide into 5 separate airtight containers and refrigerate.

11. Reheat to serve or enjoy it cold.

Chinese Pulled Pork with Mashed Cauliflower

Ingredients:

1½ pounds pork shoulder or loin

3 tablespoons tomato sauce

1 tablespoon tomato paste

¾ cup chicken stock

1 teaspoon ginger powder

1 teaspoon garlic powder

3 tablespoons soy sauce

1 teaspoon smoked paprika

1 large head cauliflower, chopped into florets

⅔ cup grated Parmesan

Chopped spring onion, to taste for garnish

Steps:

1. Place the pork in a slow cooker.

2. In a medium bowl, combine the tomato sauce, tomato paste, chicken stock, ginger powder, garlic powder, soy sauce, and paprika.

3. Pour the mixture over the pork in the slow cooker, and lift the pork to make sure mixture gets underneath.

4. Cover and cook for 7 hours on low heat.

5. Meanwhile, steam or boil the cauliflower florets until extremely tender, around 25 to 30 minutes.

6. Place the cauliflower in a large bowl with the grated Parmesan cheese and mash with a fork until it has reached a mashed-potato consistency.

7. Divide the mashed cauliflower between five airtight containers and when the pork is done, top with equal amounts of pork and refrigerate.

8. To serve, reheat and top with chopped spring onions.

Creamy Whitefish Casserole

Ingredients:

1 large head broccoli, cut into small florets
2 tablespoons oil
Salt and pepper, to taste
8 green onions, finely chopped
3 tablespoons small capers
Butter for greasing casserole dish
2 pounds whitefish, cut into 5 serving sizes
1¾ cups heavy whipping cream
2 tablespoons Dijon mustard
2 tablespoons dried parsley
3 ounces butter, sliced

Steps:

1. Preheat oven to 400°F.

2. Fry the broccoli in oil over medium-high heat until golden and soft, around 6 minutes. Season with salt and pepper. Add the green onions and capers, and continue to fry for 2 to 3 minutes.

3. Place the vegetable mixture into a butter-greased baking dish. Nestle the pieces of fish in between the vegetables.

4. In medium bowl, combine the whipping cream, mustard, and parsley, and pour the mixture over the fish and vegetables. Top with butter slices.

5. Bake until the fish is cooked through and flakes easily with a fork, around 22 minutes.

6. Divide between five airtight containers and refrigerate. Reheat to serve.

Cheesy Chicken and Broccoli Casserole

Ingredients:

1 cup cooked riced cauliflower
3 tablespoons almond meal
Your favorite seasonings
2 cups chicken broth (low sodium)
1 cup unsweetened almond milk
1 pound boneless, skinless chicken breasts, chopped into bite-size chunks
4 cups fresh broccoli florets
1½ cups of your favorite shredded cheese

Steps:

1. Preheat oven to 400°F; using extra-virgin olive oil, grease a 13 x 9 inch baking dish.

2. Add cauliflower, almond meal, your favorite seasonings, chicken broth, and milk to the dish and whisk together.

3. Add the chicken and broccoli, stirring to distribute into an even layer. Cover and bake for 20 minutes.

4. Add the cheese to the casserole and stir well to combine; return to the oven for 20 minutes, uncovered.

5. Stir and cook 20 minutes more until chicken is cooked through (total baking time is 1 hour).

Meatloaf Muffins

Ingredients:

2 eggs
½ red bell pepper, diced
½ green bell pepper, diced
½ onion, diced
1½ pounds ground turkey,
   bison, or lean beef
½ cup tomato sauce
¾ cup almond meal
1 teaspoon garlic powder
Salt and pepper, to taste
½ tablespoon extra-virgin
   olive oil to grease muffin
   tins

Steps:

1. In a large bowl, combine eggs, bell peppers, and onion. Add ground meat, tomato sauce, almond meal, garlic powder, salt, and pepper; mix well with your hands until thoroughly combined.

2. Separate meatloaf mixture and place into 12 greased muffin tins and bake for 20 minutes or until meatloaf is done and passes the toothpick test.

We hope you have found this batch-cooking chapter helpful—while some prefer to make simple meals every single day, others prefer to cook in batches and being prepared with food that is ready to go can really help keep you on track for success. Keep in mind, this was just a sample batch-cooking plan—there are several more batch-cooking recipes found in chapters 19 and 20 if you would like to create your personalized menu.

Chapter 11

Food Groups and Servings

The types of calories you consume are just as (if not more) important than the amounts of calories you consume. Due to their macro- and micronutrient contents, the following food groups are essential for weight loss, even blood sugar levels, and overall well-being, so we highly recommend making these guidelines an everyday goal to fulfill. It is important to note that you are *not* restricted to the foods listed on the next few pages—these food groups should take priority in your daily keto regimen, however, you will be able to incorporate other foods as well. For a complete list of acceptable 30-day keto foods, please refer to chapter 4.

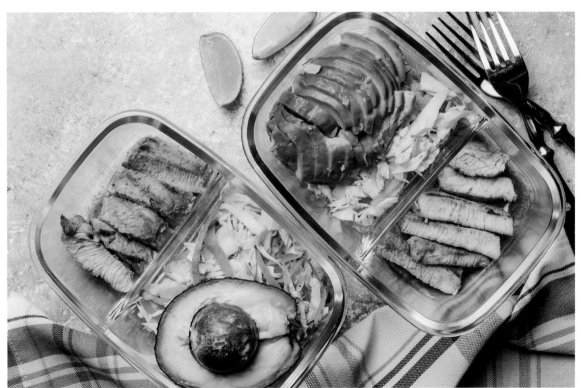

(1) Low-Glycemic Vegetables (2 to 3 servings)

Nutrient-dense vegetables are a good source of low-glycemic carbohydrates that will give you energy but help maintain even blood sugar levels. Several vitamins, such as vitamins A and C, and minerals such as iron and magnesium, are also found in these vegetables; plus many are high in calcium and fiber! If you do not see your favorite low-glycemic vegetable below, feel free to include it in your daily food regimen. The average amount of calories, carbohydrates, protein, fat, and fiber for the vegetables we provided are 12 calories, 2 grams of carbohydrates, 1 gram of protein, 0 grams of fat, and 2 grams of fiber in case you would like to compare your vegetable of choice to the ones in the recommended list.

Green Vegetable	Serving Size	Calories	Carbohydrates (grams)	Protein (grams)	Fat (grams)	Fiber (grams)
Spinach (cooked)	½ cup	23	4	3	0	2.5
Broccoli	½ cup	16	3	1.5	0	1
Kale	½ cup	17	3	1.5	0	1
Collard greens	½ cup	6	1	0.5	0	0.5
Cabbage	½ cup	9	2	0.5	0	1
Brussels sprouts	½ cup	19	4	1.5	0	1.5
Bok choy	½ cup	5	1	0.5	0	0
Romaine lettuce	½ cup	8	0.5	0.5	0	0
Arugula	½ cup	3	0	0	0	0
Cauliflower	½ cup	13	2.5	1	0	1

Earlier, we suggested two to three servings of low-glycemic vegetables per day. Whether you eat two or three servings will be based on your personal caloric needs. Since everyone is different, you can tailor your green vegetable needs based on your overall caloric intake requirements, as well as the keto macronutrient percentages you are targeting each day, given the amount of other consumed foods.

② Low-Sugar Nonfatty Fruits (0 to 2 servings)

Low-sugar fruits are another source of carbohydrates and energy. In addition, they provide even more micronutrients to add to the variety of benefits the low-glycemic vegetables boast. Try to incorporate tomato or red bell pepper in your servings of low-sugar fruits as they contain lycopene—lycopene is a powerful antioxidant that is beneficial for heart health, sun protection, and reduced risk of certain cancers. Do not have more than one serving of berries per day in order to stick to your carbohydrate requirements. Please stick to the 30-day keto low-sugar fruit choices as the selections we have handpicked for you are the lowest in sugar, and remaining extremely low in sugar will be most advantageous for reaching your goals. The average amount of calories, carbohydrates, protein, fat, and fiber for the fruits we provided are 27 calories, 6.5 grams of carbohydrates, 1 gram of protein, 0 grams of fat, and 2 grams of fiber.

Low-Sugar Fruit	Serving Size	Calories	Carbohydrates (grams)	Protein (grams)	Fat (grams)	Fiber (grams)
Tomato	½ cup	16	3.5	1	0	1
Bell pepper	½ cup	15	3.5	0	0	1
Blueberries	½ cup	43	11	0.5	0	2
Raspberries	½ cup	33	8	1	0	4
Strawberries	½ cup	25	6	0.5	0	1.5
Blackberries	½ cup	31	7	1	0	4

Earlier, we suggested to eat one to two servings of low-sugar fruits per day. Whether you eat one or two servings will be based on your personal caloric needs. Since everyone is different, you can tailor your low-sugar fruit needs based on your overall caloric intake requirements.

③ Summer and Winter Squash (0 to 1 serving)

Squash is mistakenly known as a vegetable or tuber, but it's actually a fruit, and it is another source of carbohydrates that contain essential nutrients and antioxidants. Since the keto protocol requires us to remain extremely low in carbohydrates and sugar, it is important to note the lower-carbohydrate variety of squash, which is the summer squash (zucchini, Zephyr, and cousa) however, Zephyr and cousa can be hard to find in some grocery stores. Up to two servings per day are allowed for these varieties and up to one serving per day is allowed of the winter varieties (butternut squash, pumpkin, spaghetti squash, and acorn squash). Please stick to the choices below, as other starches are too high in carbohydrates for the 30-day keto regimen. The average amount of calories, carbohydrates, protein, fat, and fiber for the starches we provided are 24 calories, 6 grams of carbohydrates, 1 gram of protein, 0 grams of fat, and 1 gram of fiber.

Squash Fruits	Serving Size	Calories	Carbohydrates (grams)	Protein (grams)	Fat (grams)	Fiber (grams)
Zucchini	1 cup	21	4	1.5	0.5	1
Zephyr	1 cup	19	4	1.5	0	1
Cousa	1 cup	20	4	1.5	0.5	1
Butternut squash	½ cup	32	8	1	0	1.5
Pumpkin	½ cup	15	4	0.5	0	0
Spaghetti squash	1 cup	31	7	1	1	1.5
Acorn squash	½ cup	28	8	0.5	0	1

Earlier, we suggested eating zero to one serving of squash fruits per day. Whether you eat zero or one serving will be based on your personal caloric needs, as well as the amount of other carbohydrates you have eaten or will plan to eat on the same day. Since everyone is different, you can tailor your squash needs based on your overall caloric intake requirements.

④ Protein (3 to 5 servings)

Protein contains amino acids, which are the essential building blocks of muscle. Muscle burns fat, but not all proteins are created equal. It is imperative to consume high-quality proteins (organic, grass-fed, and wild if possible) that are unprocessed and have minimal preservatives, fillers, and environmental toxins. If you do not see your favorite protein below, feel free to include it in your daily food regimen. The average amount of calories, carbohydrates, protein, fat, and fiber for the proteins we provided are 116 calories, .5 grams of carbohydrates, 19 grams of protein, 4 grams of fat, and 0 grams of fiber, in case you would like to compare your protein choice to the ones in the recommended list.

Protein	Serving Size	Calories	Carbohydrates (grams)	Protein (grams)	Fat (grams)	Fiber (grams)
Eggs	1 whole egg (large)	78	0.5	6	5	0
Chicken (boneless/skinless)	3 ounces	90	0	17	1.5	0
Turkey (boneless/skinless)	3 ounces	120	0	26	1	0
Cod	3 ounces	70	0	15	1	0
Shrimp	3 ounces	90	1	17	1.5	0
Scallops	3 ounces	90	5	17	0.5	0
Wild salmon	3 ounces	143	0	18	8	0
Lean beef	3 ounces	158	0	26	5	0
Chicken with skin	3 ounces	190	0	20	11	0
Turkey with skin	3 ounces	129	0	24	3	0
Canned tuna (packed in water)	3 ounces	90	0	20	1	0
Boneless pork chops	3 ounces	115	0	20	4	0
Bone-in pork chops	3 ounces	150	0	17	7	0

Earlier, we suggested eating three to five servings of protein per day. Since everyone is different, you can tailor your protein needs based on your overall caloric intake requirements. If you add your own protein to the list, be sure to avoid low-quality choices that have detrimental additives such as nitrates; items such as hot dogs, deli meats, and fast-food meats should be eliminated or severely limited.

(5) Fats (8 to 12 servings)

This group contains the beneficial fats that include properties that assist with weight loss, increasing good cholesterol, reducing bad cholesterol, and maintaining even blood sugar levels. The average amount of calories, carbohydrates, protein, fat, and fiber for the healthy fats below are 116 calories, 1.5 grams of carbohydrates, 5 grams of protein, 11 grams of fat, and 1 gram of fiber.

Fatty Food	Serving Size	Calories	Carbohydrates (grams)	Protein (grams)	Fat (grams)	Fiber (grams)
Avocado	½ cup	117	6	1.5	11	5
Walnuts	14 halves	185	4	4	18	2
Wild salmon	3 ounces	143	0	18	8	0
Eggs	1 whole egg (large)	78	0.5	6	5	0
Extra-virgin olive oil	1 tablespoon	119	0	0	14	0
Coconut oil	1 tablespoon	121	0	0	14	0
Avocado oil	1 tablespoon	124	0	0	14	0
Macadamia nuts	1 ounce	204	4	2	21	2.5
Brazil nuts	1 ounce	186	3.5	4	19	2
Fatty cuts of meat	3 ounces	158	0	26	15	0
Cream	1 tablespoon	29	0.5	0.5	3	0
Coconut milk	2 tablespoons	68	2	1	7	1
Olives	1 ounce	41	1	0	4	1
Cheddar cheese	1 ounce	113	0.5	7	9	0
Mozzarella cheese	1 ounce	78	1	8	5	0
Cottage cheese	½ cup	111	4	12	5	0
Grass-fed butter	1 tablespoon	100	0	0	11	0

Earlier, we suggested to eat eight to twelve servings of fats per day. Whether you eat eight, nine, ten, eleven, or twelve servings per day will be based on your personal caloric needs, as well as the amounts of macronutrients consumed from other foods. Since everyone is different, you can tailor your healthy fat needs based on your overall caloric intake requirements.

If you're unsure of how to incorporate these foods into a meal plan, the keto select meal planning system found in chapter 14 will detail a variety of ways to meet the above recommended requirements. For the most simplistic way to achieve these servings, you can also refer back to the Keto Meal Planning Kit in chapter 1. If you want to get even more creative, the 30-day keto breakfast, lunch, and dinner recipes found in chapters 18, 19, and 20 include a variety of these foods, incorporated into delicious meals.

Chapter 12

The Plateau Solution—Keto with Intermittent Fasting

If you follow the proper caloric intake and macronutrients accurately, you should not hit a plateau, but it can happen. A plateau is when your weight-loss results become stagnant for more than a few days. If you run into this issue, it's time to change it up and to reassess your nutrition plan.

If you do hit a plateau, before making any drastic changes, fully assess how you have been eating for the past week. If you have been truly sticking to the 30-day keto plan, the next step is to track every single calorie, gram of carbohydrate, fat, protein, and sugar that goes into your body. You may find that perhaps your nutrition plan hasn't been as targeted as you assumed. If it has been perfectly accurate in terms of carbohydrates, fats, and proteins, you may require fewer calories to achieve your ideal weight. If that's the case, try lowering your caloric intake by 300 to 500 calories per day and adjust your macronutrients (fat, carbs, protein) to fall into alignment with 70 to 80 percent fat, 10 to 20 percent protein, and 5 to 10 percent carbohydrates with your new/lower calories as a guide.

If you're certain your nutrition plan doesn't need tweaking and you're just in a genuine plateau that your body won't snap out of, we would like you to try the solution found in this chapter, which is a very strict five-day keto plan paired with intermittent fasting. Intermittent fasting is a general term for various meal planning schedules that cycle between voluntary fasting and non-fasting over a recurring time period. Intermittent fasting is complementary to the keto nutrition plan as ketones (the fuel we use to turn the gut into a fat-burning machine) are increased during fasting. Also, when you are given a certain "feeding window," lower calorie consumption may naturally occur, which can be an easy way to break a plateau. Studies and human trials do suggest that intermittent fasting may have beneficial effects on weight, body composition, cardiovascular bio-markers, and aging. At the cellular level, intermittent fasting may also increase resistance against oxidative stress, decrease inflammation, and promote longevity.[1]

There are several ways to employ intermittent fasting, so you should be able to find something doable here. Below are five popular intermittent fasting schedules:

- **16/8 Method:** This involves fasting every day for sixteen hours, allowing food and beverage consumption (besides water) for only eight hours.
- **5/2 Method:** This involves eating a normal schedule of food for five days per week with no fasting on those days. The other two days per week will be restricted to 500 calories for women and 600 calories for men.
- **Eat Stop Eat**: This involves eating normally with no fasting for two days and then eating nothing for twenty-four hours and repeating that pattern.
- **Alternate-Day Fasting:** This involves eating normally one day with no fasting and then eating only a few hundred calories the next day, repeating that pattern.
- **Spontaneous Meal Skipping:** This involves skipping at least one meal per day, not in any given pattern.

Given the 30-day keto plan, our preferred method of fasting is the 16/8 method because most of the fast takes place during sleeping hours, making it more realistic for people to achieve. We don't prefer any measures which include not eating for a full day or eating very little, as that can lead to an unhealthy relationship with food, in addition to feeling so hungry that a binge could easily happen.

So you can really shake things up and get off this plateau you may be experiencing, we have put together a very strict five-day keto plan below that falls in the lines of the 16/8 intermittent fasting method, meaning you will have an eight-hour feeding window. Another approach is that you try the 16/8 method first along with the keto foods you have been consuming already. If that doesn't break your plateau, pair the 16/8 method with the following nutrition plan.

---

1   Mary-Catherine Stockman et al., "Intermittent Fasting: Is the Wait Worth the Weight?," June 2018, ncbi.nlm.nih.gov/pmc /articles/PMC5959807/.

Your five-day sample intermittent-fasting meal plan does not include calories or portion sizes—please adjust portions based on your calorie needs. Also, keep in mind that the following plan is a guide of suggestions; if you dislike a selection of food or have an allergy, please do not consume that particular food—just make a reasonable substitution. If there are particular meals or snacks you prefer, you can use them more than once and omit others.

16/8 Intermittent Fasting Keto Schedule
8-Hour Feeding Window: 10:00 a.m.-6:00 p.m. (feel free to adjust as long as the window is eight hours, such as 11:00 a.m.-7:00 p.m. or 9:00 a.m. to 5:00 p.m.)

Day 1

Before 10:00 a.m.: Any beverage with no calories such as water, plain tea, or black coffee.

10:00 a.m. Breakfast: Coffee with cream, butter, or ghee (optional), scrambled eggs topped with cheese and avocado slices.

12:00 p.m. Snack (optional): Celery and nut butter.

1:30 p.m. Lunch: Leafy green salad topped with 2 tablespoons olive oil, vinegar, canned tuna, diced red onion, and tomatoes.

3:00 p.m. Snack (optional): Olives.

6:00 p.m. Dinner: Chicken leg (with skin), zucchini cooked with olive oil, steamed cauliflower mashed with grated Parmesan cheese.

After Dinner: Any beverage with no calories such as water, plain tea, and black coffee.

Day 2

Before 10:00 a.m.: Any beverage with no calories such as water, plain tea, and black coffee.

10:00 a.m. Breakfast: Chia pudding: mix ½ cup unsweetened coconut milk, 1½ tablespoons chia seeds, ½ teaspoon vanilla extract in a small bowl and refrigerate ahead of time, overnight or at least for one hour prior to eating. Top with berries (optional).

12:00 p.m. Snack (optional): Piece of cheese.

1:30 p.m. Lunch: Chicken tenderloins pan-fried in oil and seasonings with trio of dips: mashed avocado, mayonnaise, and Tzatziki Dipping Sauce (page 265).

3:00 p.m. Snack (optional): ¼ cup macadamia nuts or pecans.

6:00 p.m. Dinner: Steak topped with sautéed mushrooms and onions (use avocado oil or butter, white wine, garlic, and favorite seasonings to sauté), and side of roasted broccoli topped with oil, seasonings, and fresh lemon.

After Dinner: Any beverage with no calories such as water, plain tea, or black coffee.

Day 3

Before 10:00 a.m.: Any beverage with no calories such as water, plain tea, or black coffee.

10:00 a.m. Breakfast: Cottage cheese with berries and hemp seeds (optional). Coffee with cream, butter, or ghee (optional).

12:00 p.m. Snack (optional): ¼ cup macadamia nuts or pecans.

1:30 p.m. Lunch: Egg salad in lettuce cups: Combine 2–3 diced hard-boiled eggs, diced celery, diced red onion, 2 tablespoons mayo, teaspoon of mustard, salt, pepper, and diced pickle (optional). Serve in lettuce cups or over a bed of greens.

3:00 p.m. Snack (optional): Salami slices with cream cheese and sliced pickles.

6:00 p.m. Dinner: Salmon pan-cooked in butter and seasonings, paired with brussels sprouts roasted in oil and seasonings.

After Dinner: Any beverage with no calories such as water, plain tea, and black coffee.

Day 4

Before 10:00 a.m.: Any beverage with no calories such as water, plain tea, and black coffee.

10:00 a.m. Breakfast: Smoked salmon rolled up with cream cheese and diced onion, paired with sliced tomatoes. Coffee with cream, butter, or ghee (optional).

12:00 p.m. Snack (optional): Celery sticks or endive leaves dipped in mashed avocado.

1:30 p.m. Lunch: Egg salad in lettuce cups: Combine 2–3 diced hard-boiled eggs, diced celery, diced red onion, 2 tablespoons mayo, teaspoon of mustard, salt, pepper, and diced pickle (optional). Serve in lettuce cups or over a bed of greens.

3:00 p.m. Snack (optional): Salami slices with cream cheese and sliced pickles.

6:00 p.m. Dinner: Bun-less cheeseburger topped with cheese, mayo, mustard, onion, and tomato with side of Parmesan roasted zucchini.

After Dinner: Any beverage with no calories such as water, plain tea, or black coffee.

Day 5

Before 10:00 a.m.: Any beverage with no calories such as water, plain tea, and black coffee.

10:00 a.m. Breakfast: Traditional bacon and eggs with side of berries. Coffee with cream, butter, or ghee (optional).

12:00 p.m. Snack (optional): Piece of cheese.

1:30 p.m. Lunch: Cobb salad with chicken or turkey, crumbled cheese, onion, tomato, avocado, and bacon.

3:00 p.m. Snack (optional): 2–3 squares dark chocolate dipped in peanut butter.

6:00 p.m. Dinner: Grilled pork chops paired with sauerkraut.

After Dinner: Any beverage with no calories such as water, plain tea, and black coffee.

Remember to make a note of your plateaued weight before starting this regimented five-day intermittent fasting plan as you should see results in five days (or less). If this plan works for you, feel free to continue it, as there is no danger in this type of intermittent fasting schedule. You can simply stick to your eight-hour feeding window while incorporating your preferred 30-day keto plan foods.

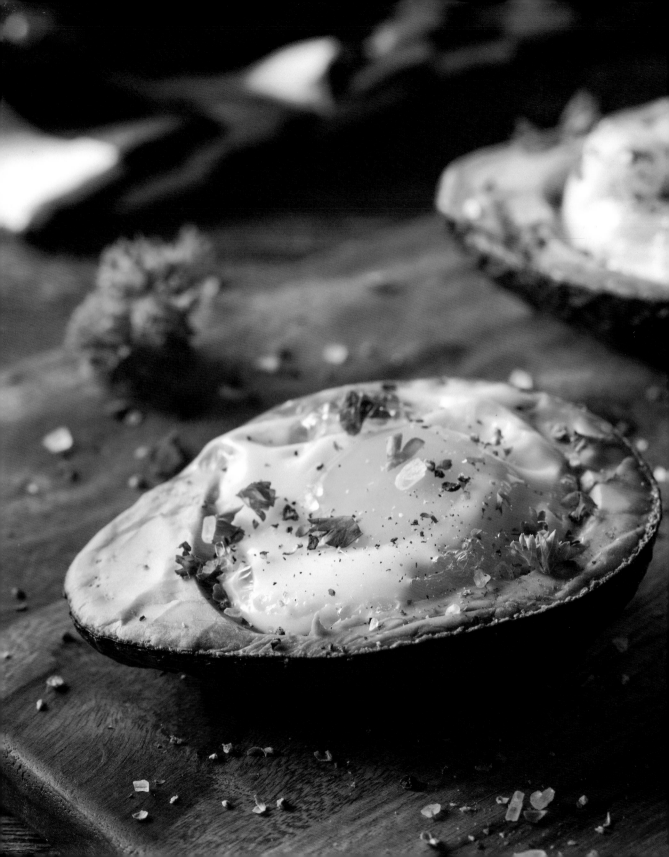

Chapter 13

Where Do My Keto Nutrients Come From?

Adhering to the 30-day keto plan does not mean you'll be missing out on vital vitamins and minerals, as proper nutrients are plentiful when choosing the appropriate keto foods. Avoiding high-glycemic and high-starch carbohydrates such as bread, pasta, cereal, rice, and potatoes does not have to mean missing out on vitamins, minerals, and fiber as there is an array of those nutrients in other foods, despite the popular misconception that you need fortified processed foods to meet your micronutrient intake. You will find a variety of charts and tables in this chapter that will serve as a handy reference for you to quickly find the nutrients you're looking for, a general guideline of how much you should consume on a daily basis, and the corresponding foods that boast each nutrient.

Mainstream dietary recommendations are strongly influenced by lobbying, funding, and food manufacturers, so when these types of vitamin and mineral charts are found on our governmental websites, the food source recommendations are comprised heavily of big-name processed foods that have fortified synthetic nutrients. Many of those foods consist of high-glycemic selections such as fortified juices, cereals, and breads, as well as other unhealthy foods such as margarine and vegetable oil. We must ponder these recommendations, and question them being based on nutrition science and truth, as opposed to funding from special interest groups. The following 30-day keto plan macro- and micronutrient charts contain unprocessed, whole foods that have naturally occurring vitamins and minerals.

Vitamins

Vitamin	Function	Food Source	Daily Amount
Biotin	Metabolizes protein, fat, carbohydrates for energy; beneficial for skin, hair, and nail health	Avocado, cauliflower, eggs, liver, pecans, pork, raspberries, salmon, sunflower seeds, walnuts	300 mcg
Folate	Metabolizes protein and assists with red blood cell formation; prevents birth defects (pregnant women should consume 600–800 mcg per day)	Arugula, asparagus, avocado, beef liver, broccoli, brussels sprouts, eggs, flaxseeds, kale, lemon, lime, walnuts	400 mcg
Niacin	Aids with nervous system functioning and digestion; helps convert food into energy.	Anchovies, avocado, chicken breast, ground beef, liver, mushrooms, peanut butter, pork, salmon, tuna, turkey	20 mg
Pantothenic Acid	Helps the functioning of the nervous system and formation of red blood cells; metabolizes fat and aids in hormone production	Avocados, broccoli, eggs, cauliflower, portobello mushrooms, poultry, salmon, sunflower seeds, yogurt	10 mg
Riboflavin	Assists with general growth and development, red blood cell formation, and energy conversion from foods	Almonds, beef liver, eggs, lamb, mushrooms, oysters, poultry, spinach, tahini, wild salmon, yogurt	1.7 mg
Thiamine	Converts food to energy and assists with nervous system functioning	Asparagus, brussels sprouts, beef liver, nutritional yeast, macadamia nuts, pork, sunflower seeds, seaweed	1.5 mg
Vitamin A	Beneficial for vision, immune function, and reproduction; assists with growth and development, as well as red blood cell, skin, and bone formation	Broccoli, beef liver, butter, collard greens, eggs, goat cheese, kale, red peppers, romaine lettuce, salmon, spinach, trout	5,000 IU

Vitamin B6	Assists with nervous system, immune function, and red blood cell formation; helps metabolize protein, fat, and carbohydrates	Avocado, chicken, eggs, nutritional yeast, pork, ricotta cheese, salmon, tuna, turkey, spinach	2 mg
Vitamin B12	Helps convert food into energy, and assists with red blood cell formation and nervous system function	Beef, clams, eggs, nutritional yeast, sardines, salmon, seaweed, trout, tuna, yogurt	6 mcg
Vitamin C	Assists with immune function and wound healing; combats free radicals, and helps with collagen and connective tissue formation	Broccoli, brussels sprouts, bell peppers, berries, lemon, lime, tomatoes	60 mg
Vitamin D	Regulates blood pressure and balances calcium; promotes hormone production, bone growth, immune and nervous system function	Beef liver, egg yolks, herring, oysters, salmon, sardines, shrimp, tuna, responsible sun exposure	1,000 - 4,000 IU
Vitamin E	Strong antioxidant to combat free radicals; Supports immune function and blood vessel formation	Almonds, avocado, Brazil nuts, broccoli, hazelnuts, peanut butter, pine nuts, rainbow trout, red sweet pepper, salmon, spinach, sunflower seeds	30 IU
Vitamin K	Supports strong bones and aids blood clotting	Avocado, blackberries, blueberries, broccoli, brussels sprouts, cabbage, cauliflower, collard greens, kale, mustard greens, spinach, Swiss chard, turnip greens	80 mcg

Minerals

Mineral	Function	Food Source	Daily Amount
Calcium	Supports nervous system and promotes bone and teeth formation; assists with blood clotting, muscle contraction, and hormone secretion, as well as constriction and relaxation of blood vessels	Almonds, broccoli, canned salmon, cheese, cottage cheese, fresh salmon, Greek yogurt, kale, sardines, sesame seeds, spinach, turnip greens	1,000 mg
Chloride	Converts food into energy, and aids digestion and fluid balance; promotes acid-base balance and nervous system function	Celery, lettuce, olives, seaweed, sea salt, tomatoes	3,400 mg
Chromium	Promotes protein, fat, and carbohydrate metabolism, and supports insulin function	Basil, beef, broccoli, garlic, green beans, romaine lettuce, turkey	120 mcg
Copper	Promotes bone, collagen, and connective tissue formation; assists with iron metabolism, energy production, and nervous system function; antioxidant that combats free radicals	Almonds, dark chocolate, kale, liver, lobster, oysters, sesame seeds, shitake mushrooms, spinach, spirulina, Swiss chard	2 mg
Iodine	Supports thyroid hormone production, reproduction, and metabolism; promotes general growth and development	Cod, cottage cheese, eggs, Greek yogurt, green beans, kale, seaweed, shrimp, strawberries, tuna, turkey	150 mcg
Iron	Promotes growth and development, immune function, and energy production; assists with red blood cell production, and wound healing, as well as the reproductive system	Beef, broccoli, clams, collard greens, dark chocolate, liver, mussels, oysters, pine nuts, pistachios, pumpkin seeds, spinach, Swiss chard, turkey	18 mg
Magnesium	Assists with blood pressure and blood sugar regulation, as well as heart rhythm stabilization; promotes immune function, bone formation, energy production, and hormone secretion; strengthens nervous system function, muscle contraction, and protein formation	Almonds, avocado, Brazil nuts, chia seeds, collard greens, dark chocolate, flax seeds, halibut, kale, mackerel, pumpkin seeds, salmon, spinach	400 mg

Manganese	Promotes cartilage and bone formation, as well as wound healing; assists with cholesterol, carbohydrate, and protein metabolism	Almonds, black tea, collard greens, green tea, kale, mussels, pecans, pine nuts, raspberries, spinach, strawberries	2 mg
Molybdenum	Promotes enzyme production	Almonds, bell pepper, celery, cod, cucumber, cheese, eggs, fennel, Greek yogurt, liver, tomatoes, romaine lettuce, sesame seeds, walnuts	75 mcg
Phosphorus	Promotes hormone activation, energy storage and production, and bone formation; supports acid-base balance	Brazil nuts, carp, cheese, chicken, clams, cottage cheese, liver, pine nuts, pistachios, pollack, pork, pumpkin seeds, salmon, sardines, scallops, sunflower seeds, turkey, yogurt	1,000 mg
Potassium	Supports heart function, blood pressure regulation, fluid balance, and nervous system function; promotes general growth and development, muscle contraction, protein formation, and carbohydrate metabolism	Artichoke, avocado, broccoli, brussels sprouts, butternut squash, clams, haddock, pumpkin seeds, salmon, spinach, sunflower seeds, Swiss chard, tomatoes, yogurt	3,500 mg
Selenium	Supports thyroid and immune function, as well as reproduction; antioxidant that fights off free radicals	Beef, Brazil nuts, chicken, clams, cottage cheese, crab, eggs, halibut, mushrooms, oysters, pork, salmon, sardines, shrimp, spinach, sunflower seeds, turkey, yogurt	70 mcg
Zinc	Promotes growth and development, protein formation, immune function, and wound healing; supports nervous system function and reproduction, as well as taste and smell	Almonds, beef, cheese, crab, eggs, green beans, hemp seeds, kale, pork, pumpkin seeds, lamb, mussels, oysters, pine nuts, sesame seeds, shrimp	15 mg

Now for a different perspective, below you will find micronutrients categorized by food group and macronutrient categories. Just like the above vitamin and mineral sources, these following foods are all keto-approved. The meal plans and recipes found throughout this book use these foods as primary ingredients to give you the best nutrition while hitting your 30-day keto plan requirements.

Food	Macronutrients	Micronutrients
Low-Glycemic Vegetables (broccoli, asparagus, brussels sprouts, onion, cauliflower, spinach, kale, artichoke, collard greens, arugula, butter lettuce, romaine, Swiss chard, cabbage, radish, zucchini)	Carbohydrate	Vitamins A, C, E, and K; chromium, folate, fiber, pantothenic acid, vitamins B1, B2, and B6; manganese, selenium, pantothenic acid, niacin, potassium, phosphorus, choline, copper, omega-3 fatty acids, calcium, and iron
Low-Sugar Fruits (blueberries, blackberries, raspberries, strawberries, tomato, bell pepper)	Carbohydrate	Vitamins A, C, E, and K, fiber, biotin, molybdenum, copper, potassium, riboflavin, thiamine, manganese, fiber, vitamins B2 and B6, folate, niacin, phosphorus, carotenoids
Other Low-Sugar Fruits (avocado, olives)	Fat	Vitamins C, E, and K, fiber, copper, potassium, vitamin B6, folate, omega-3 fatty acids
Nuts and Seeds (almonds, pistachios, pecans, macadamia, Brazil nuts, pine nuts, walnuts, hazelnuts, sesame seeds, pumpkin seeds, chia seeds, flax seeds)	Fat and Protein	Vitamin E, vitamins B2 and B6, magnesium, zinc, fiber, biotin, copper, phosphorus, calcium, omega-3 fatty acids
Poultry (organic chicken, duck, turkey)	Protein	Vitamins B2, B3, B6, and B12; niacin, phosphorus, choline, iron, selenium, zinc, phosphorus, choline, and pantothenic acid
Other Poultry (eggs)	Protein and Fat	Vitamins A, D, E, K; choline, vitamin B12, thiamine, riboflavin, folate, zinc, copper, and selenium
Fish (wild salmon, halibut, sole, rockfish, trout, tuna, anchovies, mahi mahi, opah, sardines)	Protein and Fat	Vitamin D, vitamins B5, B6, and B12, magnesium, potassium, niacin, phosphorus, and selenium; omega-3 fatty acids
Shellfish (oysters, clams, shrimp, mussels, crab, lobster)	Protein and Fat	Vitamin B12, iron, zinc, copper, omega-3 fatty acids
Meat (organic grass-fed beef, organic grass-fed lamb, venison, bison)	Protein and Fat	Vitamins B3, B6, and B12; omega-3 fatty acids, selenium, iron, zinc, phosphorus, choline, and pantothenic acid
Dairy (Greek yogurt, cheese, cottage cheese)	Protein and Fat	Probiotics, calcium, potassium, vitamin A, vitamins B2, B6, and B12, zinc, phosphorus, selenium, and magnesium

As you can see, staple foods found in the 30-day keto plan offer an abundance of essential vitamins and minerals, despite the fact that many dietary recommendations suggest processed foods due to their synthetic nutrient composition. Some processed foods do, in fact, offer fortified vitamins and minerals, however, one can find several whole foods that offer naturally occurring nutrients with superior absorption rates. As an added benefit, when consuming the above-mentioned whole foods as opposed to fortified breads, cereals, pastas, and fruit juices, you will avoid high-glycemic carbohydrates that contribute to raised blood sugar levels and potential weight gain.

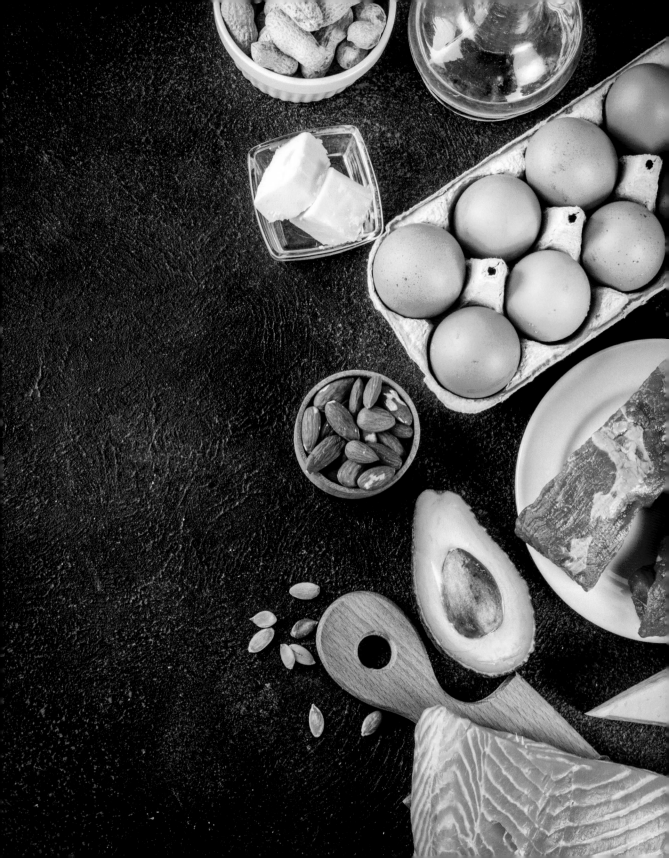

Chapter 14

The "Keto Select" Meal Planning System

T he keto select meal planning system is your simplistic guide to daily food recommendations that can be used when you need quick and easy ideas for breakfast, lunch, dinner, and snacks. The different categories to select from will lead the proper keto macros on your plate. You may be wondering, *do I use the keto select meal planning system or the recipes found in coming chapters?* The meal planning system in this chapter is a road map of basic food choices to follow, and it's specifically designed for those who don't have time for recipes. If you are feeling more adventurous, feel free to substitute any meal with one of the delicious recipes found in chapters 18, 19, 20, and 21.

Unlike the typical, rigid meal plan, the keto select meal planning system gives you several options for breakfast, lunch, dinner, and snacks—it's a "choose your own adventure" of sorts. At the beginning of each section are directions that explain possible food options for that particular meal or snack. This will allow for some flexibility with regard to your taste buds, how hungry you are, caloric needs, and what you have on hand. The pick-four planning system is based on simplicity, convenience, and foods that are sound with regard to overall health as well as weight loss. All meals here, as well as those in later chapters, should you choose to substitute some, provide dense nutrition, while following the guidelines of the 30-day keto plan.

The items listed in the meal planning system are easily found in most grocery stores and the majority of the instructions (we won't even call them recipes) are easy. We do not list every single keto-approved food in the meal planning system, so if are wondering about appropriate substitutions, refer back to chapter 4 to make sure your food is allowed on your 30-day keto plan.

How to Meal Plan—Breakfast

Choose one or two options from the fatty protein category, one or two from the additional fat category, and one or two selections (optional) from the low-glycemic produce category. If you select two from the low-glycemic produce section, no more than one can come from berries.

Fatty Protein

1 to 3 Eggs Your Way: Choose your favorite preparation style—boiled, poached, scrambled, over easy, or sunny-side up.

1 or 2 Eggs Your Way with Smoked Salmon, Bacon, or Sausage: Choose your favorite egg preparation style and pair with 2 to 3 ounces of smoked salmon, 2 to 3 slices of uncured, nitrate-free bacon, or 2 to 3 pieces of breakfast sausage.

Smoked Salmon: 3 to 4 ounces.

Herring: 3 to 4 ounces.

Bacon: 2 to 3 pieces.

Breakfast Sausage: 2 to 4 ounces.

Steak: 4 to 8 ounces.

Cheese: 1 to 2 ounces.

Full-Fat Cottage Cheese: ½ to 1 cup cottage cheese.

Plain Full-Fat Greek Yogurt: ½ to ⅔ cup Greek yogurt.

Plain Full-Fat Kefir: ½ to 2/3 cup kefir.

Plain Full-Fat Coconut Yogurt: ½ to ⅔ cup coconut yogurt.

Unsweetened Full-Fat Coconut Milk: ½ to ⅔ cup coconut milk.

Plain Full-Fat Almond Yogurt: ½ to ⅔ cup almond yogurt.

Additional Fat

Avocado: ½ avocado, sliced or mashed.

Olives: ¼ cup chopped olives.

Cheese: 1 slice of your favorite cheese or ¼ cup of your favorite shredded cheese, or 2 tablespoons cream cheese.

Nuts: 1 ounce almonds, pecans, pistachios, pine nuts, macadamia nuts, Brazil nuts, walnuts, or similar.

Seeds: 1 tablespoon chia seeds, flax seeds, hemp seeds, or sesame seeds.

Oils: 1 tablespoon healthy oil for sautéing.

Dairy: 1 to 2 tablespoons heavy cream, butter, or ghee.

Nondairy: 1 to 2 tablespoons coconut milk or cream.

Nut/seed butters: 1 tablespoon nut or seed butter such as peanut butter, almond butter, cashew butter, macadamia butter, or sesame butter.

Mayonnaise: 1 tablespoon avocado oil mayo or regular mayo.

Dressings & sauces: 1 or 2 tablespoons of any high-fat, low-carbohydrate, and low-sugar dressing or sauce.

Low-Glycemic Produce

Strawberries: 4 to 5 medium strawberries.

Blueberries: ½ cup blueberries.

Raspberries: ½ cup raspberries.

Blackberries: ½ cup blackberries.

Mixed berries: ½ cup mixed berries.

Tomato: ½ cup sliced tomato.

Avocado: ½ avocado, sliced or mashed.

Bell pepper: ½ cup bell pepper, sliced or diced.

Mushrooms: ½ cup mushrooms, sliced or diced.

Onions: ¼ cup onions, sliced or diced.

Spinach: 1 cup raw or ½ cup cooked.

Kale: 1 cup raw or ½ cup cooked.

Asparagus: 2 to 3 spears.

Broccoli: ½ to 1 cup cooked.

Leafy greens: 1 to 2 cups.

Omelet produce mix (onions, bell pepper, mushrooms): ½ cup.

Example Breakfast Meals
Using the Keto Select Guidelines

Keto Select Formula Sample 1:

Steak (fatty protein) +

Egg (fatty protein) +

Cooking oil (additional fat) +

Asparagus (low-glycemic produce) +

Tomato (low-glycemic produce)

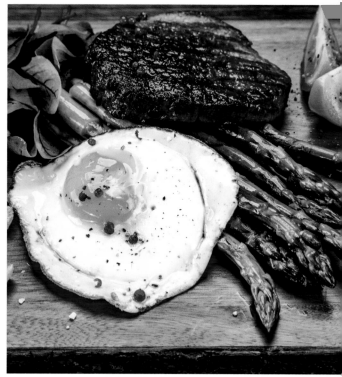

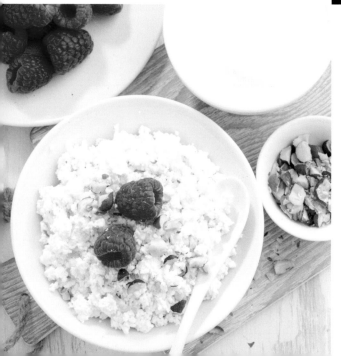

Keto Select Formula Sample 2:

Cottage cheese (fatty protein) +

Nuts (additional fat) +

Raspberries (low-glycemic produce)

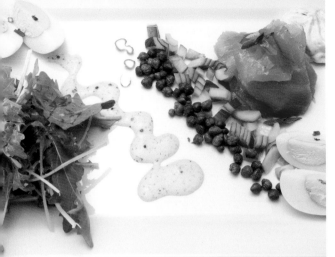

Keto Select Formula Sample 3:
Eggs (fatty protein) +
Salmon (fatty protein) +
Crème fraîche (additional fat) +
Diced onions (low-glycemic produce) +
Leafy greens (low-glycemic produce)

Keto Select Formula Sample 4:
Mushroom omelet:
Eggs (fatty protein) +
Cheese (additional fat) +
Mushrooms (low-glycemic produce) +
Sour cream (additional fat) +
Tomato (low-glycemic produce)

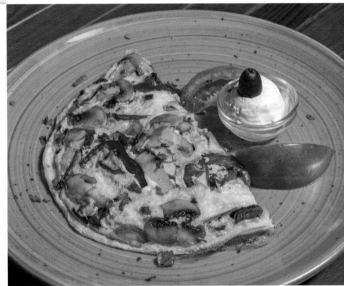

Keto Select Formula Sample 5:
Greek yogurt (fatty protein) +
Walnuts (additional fat) +
Strawberries (low-glycemic produce)

How to Meal Plan—Lunch and Dinner

Select one fatty protein or one lean protein. If you select a fatty protein, choose at least one or two additional fats. If you select a lean protein, choose at least two or three additional fats. Choose one or two selections from the low-glycemic produce category (optional).

Fatty Protein

Ground Beef: 6 to 8 ounces.

Chicken with Skin on: 6 to 8 ounces.

Turkey with Skin on: 6 to 8 ounces.

Salami: 2 to 4 ounces.

Ham: 2 to 4 ounces.

Pork Sausage: 2 to 4 ounces.

Eggs: 2 to 3 whole eggs, prepared any style.

Cheese: 1 to 2 ounces.

Fresh or Canned Salmon: 6 to 8 ounces.

Smoked Salmon: 2 to 4 ounces.

Trout: 6 to 8 ounces.

Mackerel: 6 to 8 ounces.

Catfish: 6 to 8 ounces.

Sardines: 4 to 8 ounces.

Steak (New York, Ribeye, T-Bone, Skirt, Filet Mignon): 6 to 8 ounces.

Bone-in Pork Chops or Lamb Chops: 6 to 8 ounces.

Lean Protein

Sirloin Steak: 6 to 8 ounces.

Boneless Pork Chops: 6 to 8 ounces.

Boneless, Skinless Chicken or Turkey: 6 to 8 ounces.

Deli Turkey: 2 to 4 ounces.

Turkey Sausage: 2 to 4 ounces.

Ground Turkey or Chicken: 6 to 8 ounces.

Canned Chicken or Tuna: 4 to 8 ounces.

Shrimp or Prawns: 4 to 8 ounces.

Crab, Clams, or Mussels: 4 to 6 ounces.

Snapper, Cod, Haddock, Sole, Halibut, or Swordfish: 6 to 8 ounces.

Additional Fat

Avocado: ½ avocado, sliced or mashed.

Olives: ¼ cup chopped olives.

Cheese: 1 slice of your favorite cheese or ¼ cup of your favorite shredded cheese, or 2 tablespoons cream cheese.

Nuts: 1 ounce almonds, pecans, pistachios, pine nuts, macadamia nuts, Brazil nuts, walnuts, or similar.

Seeds: 1 tablespoon chia seeds, flax seeds, hemp seeds, or sesame seeds.

Oils: 1 tablespoon healthy oil for sautéing.

Dairy: 1 tablespoon heavy cream, butter, or ghee.

Nondairy: 1 to 2 tablespoons coconut milk or cream.

Nut/Seed Butters: 1 tablespoon nut or seed butter such as peanut butter, almond butter, cashew butter, macadamia butter, or sesame butter.

Bacon: 1 to 2 strips bacon, chopped.

Mayonnaise: 1 tablespoon avocado oil mayo or regular mayo.

Dressings & Sauces: 1 or 2 tablespoons of any high-fat, low-carbohydrate, and low-sugar dressing or sauce.

Low-Glycemic Produce

Zucchini: 1 cup, cooked.

Spaghetti Squash: 1 cup, cooked.

Fennel: ½ to 1 cup, cooked.

Tomato: ½ cup sliced tomato.

Avocado: ½ avocado, sliced or mashed.

Bell Pepper: ½ cup bell pepper, diced.

Mushrooms: ½ cup mushrooms, diced.

Onions: ¼ cup onions, sliced or diced.

Hot Peppers: ½ cup, sliced.

Pickles: ½ cup, sliced.

Spinach: 1 cup raw or ½ cup, cooked.

Kale: 1 cup raw or ½ cup, cooked.

Asparagus: 3 to 4 spears.

Green Beans: 1 cup, cooked.

Broccoli: ½ to 1 cup, cooked.

Brussels Sprouts: ½ to 1 cup cooked,

Cucumber: ½ to 1 cup, sliced.

Leafy Greens: 1 to 2 cups.

Cabbage: 1 to 2 cups.

Burger Topper Combo: 2 to 3 lettuce leaves, 1 large slice tomato, 1 thin slice onion.

Small Mixed Salad: 1 to 2 cups leafy greens, ⅓ cup diced tomato/onion, ½ avocado.

Sandwich Lettuce Cup Combo: 2 to 4 large lettuce leaf cups, ⅓ cup diced tomato/onion, ½ avocado, sliced.

Mixed Produce: 1 to 2 cups any mixed low-glycemic produce.

Example Lunch and Dinner Meals Using the Keto Select Guidelines

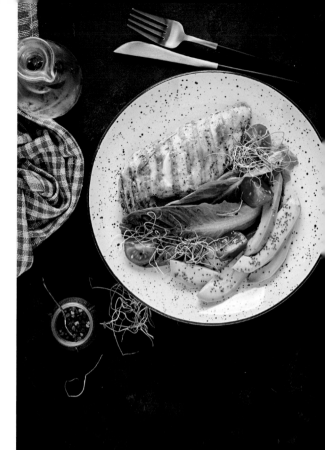

Keto Select Formula Sample 1:

Chicken (lean protein) +

Cooking oil (additional fat) +

Avocado (additional fat) +

Leafy greens (low-glycemic produce) +

Tomato (low-glycemic produce)

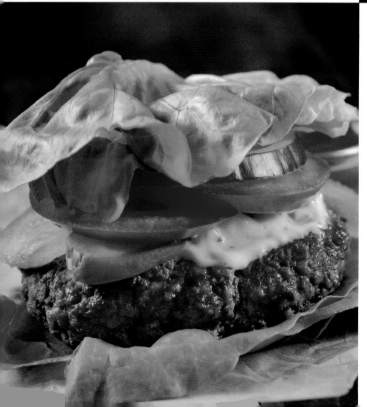

Keto Select Formula Sample 2:

Ground Beef (fatty protein) +

Mayonnaise (additional fat) +

Burger topper combo (low-glycemic produce) +

Pickles (low-glycemic produce)

Keto Select Formula Sample 3:

Shrimp (lean protein) +

Avocado (additional fat) +

Pesto (additional fat) +

Parmesan cheese (additional fat) +

Spinach (low-glycemic produce) +

Zucchini noodles (low-glycemic
produce)

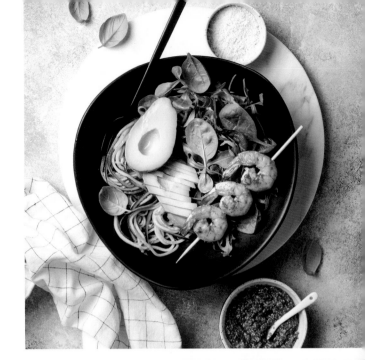

Keto Select Formula Sample 4:

Eggs (fatty protein) +

Mayonnaise (additional fat) +

Leafy greens (low-glycemic produce)

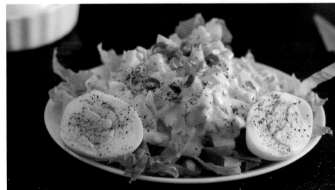

Keto Select Formula Sample 5:

Ground chicken (lean protein) +

Cooking oil (additional fat) +

Cheese (additional fat) +

Cucumber (low-glycemic produce) +

Burger topper combo (low-glycemic
produce)

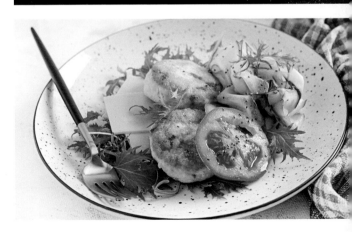

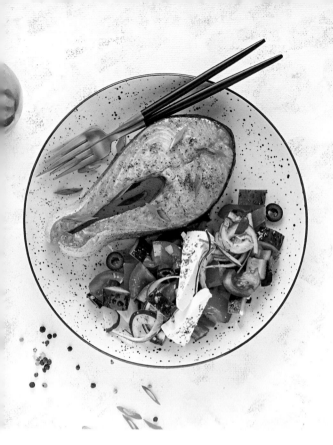

Keto Select Formula Sample 6:
Salmon (fatty protein) +
Feta cheese (additional fat) +
Olives (additional fat) +
Mixed produce (low-glycemic produce)

Keto Select Formula Sample 7:
Steak (fatty protein) +
Loaded cauliflower: cauliflower
    (low-glycemic produce) +
Cheese (additional fat) +
Bacon (additional fat) +
Asparagus (low-glycemic produce)

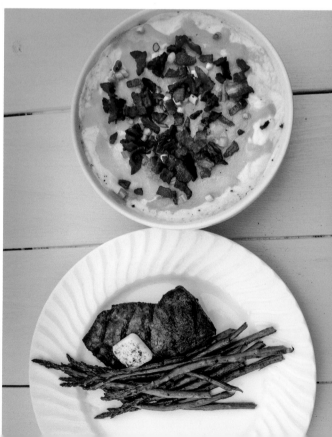

As a reminder, not all keto-approved foods are found in this chapter—please refer to chapter 4 if you're looking for additions or substitutions. The Keto Select Meal Planning System employs common, easy-to-find foods that most mainstream grocery stores carry. For a variety of unique breakfast, lunch, dinner, side dish, sauce, and dressing recipes, refer to chapters 18, 19, 20, and 21.

Chapter 15

Niche Keto Foods
to Know About

There are several foods in the ketogenic world that are quite unique and possibly even unheard of in some parts. If you haven't heard of many of the niche keto foods or are unsure of what they are used for, you are not alone. The purpose of this chapter is to outline and explain popular high-fat, low-carbohydrate, low-sugar items that may not be ones you, personally, have ever had in your grocery cart. The following list merely gives you more options that will help you achieve your 30-day keto plan macronutrient breakdown. If you are doing fine on your own with more mainstream foods, don't feel obligated to purchase or use any of the below foods. If you're looking for more options or you want to get more creative in the kitchen, you may find this chapter beneficial.

Coconut Oil

Extracted from the meat of mature coconuts, coconut oil is very popular in the keto community as its fat profile is different than most other cooking oils. Typically, fats in the diet come from long-chain triglycerides, however, the fats found in coconut oil are called medium-chain triglycerides (MCTs) as these fats are shorter, having between six and twelve carbons. There are four primary MCTs that are categorized, based on their carbon lengths—C6 (caproic acid) contains six carbons, C8 (caprylic acid) contains eight carbons, C10 (capric acid) contains ten carbons, and C12 (lauric acid) contains twelve carbons. Because of their chemical structure, MCTs go to the liver where they are used as a quick source of energy, and they can increase fat burning, as well as raise your HDL (good) cholesterol.[1] Coconut oil provides a mixture of all medium-chain triglycerides, and is most abundant in C12 (lauric acid). Once digested, lauric acid helps create mono-laurin, which in turn helps kill harmful bacteria, viruses, and fungi. [2] Coconut oil can be used for cooking at high heat, creamer for coffee, added nutrients in smoothies, and moisturizing the skin without added chemicals.

MCT Oil

The primary difference between coconut oil and MCT oil is that coconut oil is comprised of around 55 percent medium-chain triglycerides, whereas MCT oil is 100 percent medium-chain triglycerides. In addition, while C12 (lauric acid) is beneficial to fend off harmful bacteria, viruses, and fungi, it is the most prevalent MCT found in coconut oil. Since it is the longest MCT, it is the least efficient in terms of converting to ketones. For greater ketone conversion, MCT oil contains a much higher proportion of C8 (caprylic acid) and C10 (capric acid) which are known for brain health and curbing hunger. These specific MCTs will give you the benefits of a strict ketogenic nutrition plan, while allowing you to consume more carbohydrates. A 2015 meta-analysis found that MCTs helped decrease weight, hip and waist circumference, visceral fat, and total body fat.[3] MCT oil has no taste or smell and can be taken on its own or added to coffee, smoothies, and salad dressings.

Keto Coffee

Keto coffee is a high-fat, high-calorie coffee that is typically made with brewed coffee, grass-fed butter or ghee, and MCT oil. It is suggested to use a blender to thoroughly

1   Chinwong, S., D. Chinwong, and A. Mangklabruks. "Daily Consumption of Virgin Coconut Oil Increases High-Density Lipoprotein Cholesterol Levels in Healthy Volunteers: A Randomized Crossover Trial." NCBI. December 14, 2017. Accessed May 19, 2019. nlm.nih.gov/pmc/articles/PMC5745680/.

2   Kabara, J., D. Swieczkowski, A. Conley, and J. Truant. "Fatty Acids and Derivatives as Antimicrobial Agents." NCBI. July 1972. Accessed May 19, 2019. ncbi.nlm.nih.gov/pmc/articles/PMC444260/.

3   Mumme, K., and W. Stonehouse. "Effects of Medium-chain Triglycerides on Weight Loss and Body Composition: A Meta-analysis of Randomized Controlled Trials." NCBI. February 2015. Accessed May 19, 2019. ncbi.nlm.nih.gov/pubmed/25636220.

combine the ingredients for a smooth and frothy texture. Since keto coffee does offer a substantial amount of fat and calories, some choose to use the coffee as a breakfast replacement. For a simple keto coffee recipe, see page 185.

Dark Chocolate

Dark chocolate is an acceptable keto dessert or snack as it is high in fat, while remaining low in sugar. Be sure to choose a minimum of 75 percent cocoa solids, as the higher the cocoa content, the lower the sugar. One glass of red wine has one to two grams of sugar so the pairing of dark chocolate with your favorite cabernet will make the perfect 30-day keto plan dessert.

Seaweed

Seaweed is a less commonly consumed vegetable, and it is one of the best vegan sources of omega-3 fatty acids. Seaweed and other marine algae actually have even more concentrated vitamins and minerals compared to vegetables that are grown on land. An excellent source of vitamin K, B, zinc and iron, as well as antioxidants, seaweed can be eaten on its own, as a side dish, or in salads.

Hemp Seeds

Hemp seeds have a very mild nutty flavor and almost go unnoticed when added to dishes as they are so subtle, with a delicate (non-crunchy) texture. Three tablespoons of hemp seeds boast 15 grams of fat, many of which come from omega-3 fatty acids. They are also an excellent source of iron, thiamine, phosphorus, magnesium, and manganese. You can sprinkle hemp seeds on salads, yogurt, or in smoothies.

Ground Psyllium Husk Powder

Psyllium is a type of fiber that is formed from the husks of the *Plantago ovata* plant's seeds. A natural laxative, many studies show that taking this supplement is beneficial for digestion, as well as heart and pancreas health. The powder is gluten-free and low carbohydrate and is used for keto baking. The psyllium husk acts like a binder and helps keto-friendly breads have the same type of texture and consistency as traditional baked goods. This ingredient is a staple in keto baking as it causes bread to hold more moisture and achieve a light, airy consistency.

Coconut Flour

Coconut flour is a naturally grain-free and gluten-free flour that is made from dried coconut meat—coconut milk production results in the by-product of coconut flour. Rich in medium-chain triglycerides, it can help you achieve and maintain ketosis, and also promotes good digestion, heart health, and stable blood sugar. High in protein and fiber, while remaining low in carbohydrates, coconut flour is popular in the keto and paleo communities for baking.

Shirataki Noodles

Shirataki are thin and translucent traditional Japanese noodles made from glucomannan, a fiber that comes from the root of the konjac plant. Shirataki are comprised of 97 percent water and 3 percent glucomannan; many studies suggest that glucomannan is associated with weight loss, as well as the reduction of body fat and cholesterol.[4] Besides noodles made from squash and zucchini, these are the only true pasta-like noodles that are acceptable in the keto and paleo communities, as they are low in calories and carbohydrates while still high in fiber.

Nutritional Yeast

Nutritional yeast is a deactivated yeast with a cheesy flavor, found in flake or powder form. It is vegan-friendly and a substantial source of fiber, amino acids, and vitamin B12. Since it is very low in carbohydrates and sugar, it makes the perfect addition to the keto nutrition plan, especially if one is dairy-free. Sprinkled on salads and entrées for added

---

4   Kaats, GR, D. Bagchi, and HG Preuss. "Konjac Glucomannan Dietary Supplementation Causes Significant Fat Loss in Compliant Overweight Adults." NCBI. October 22, 2015. Accessed May 20, 2019. ncbi.nlm.nih.gov/pubmed/26492494.

savory flavor, or made into a plant-based cheese sauce (see page 267), it makes a wonderful addition to most dishes.

Tahini

Tahini is a creamy nondairy butter that is made strictly from sesame seeds. In addition to being plant-based, tahini is high in healthy fats, moderate in protein and fiber, and low in carbohydrates. It's also packed with nutrients including copper, manganese, calcium, magnesium, iron, zinc, selenium, and thiamine. Tahini can be used in dips, sauces, smoothies, and salad dressing, or alone as a seed butter—see page 271 for a creamy tahini dressing recipe.

Ghee

Ghee is clarified butter that is made from heating butter, which separates the liquid and milk portions from the fat. The milk turns into a solid, and the remaining oil is ghee. Since the milk separates from the oil, ghee is dairy-free and has a much higher smoke point than butter. Ghee can be melted over vegetables, used in keto coffee (page 185), or used in place of oil or butter when cooking dishes such as stir-fry or eggs.

Bone Broth

Bone broth is made by simmering the bones and connective tissues of beef, pork, lamb, turkey, chicken, bison, venison, or fish. It is more nutrient-dense than standard broth and stock due to its longer cooking time, however, the nutrient content is determined by the bones used in the broth. Animal bones are packed with calcium, magnesium, potassium, and phosphorus, whereas fish bones also contain iodine, which is important for metabolism and thyroid function. Connective tissues provide glucosamine and chondroitin which support joint health, and marrow supplies vitamin A, vitamin K2, zinc, iron, boron, manganese, and selenium, as well as omega-3 fatty acids. The above-mentioned components also contain the protein collagen, which turns into gelatin when cooked and produces numerous essential amino acids. As the ingredients simmer, the water absorbs the nutrients, so the vitamins and minerals can be consumed via drinking bone broth on its own or from incorporating it in soups, sauces, and gravies.

Avocado Oil Mayo

Regular mayonnaise can be used in your keto nutrition plan, however, avocado oil mayo (or sometimes called "paleo mayo") has a healthier fat composition due to the fact that avocado oil is superior to the oils used in standard commercial mayonnaise. Avocado oil mayo is higher in monounsaturated fats and extremely low in sugar and carbohydrates—it can be pricey in some grocery stores, so please refer to page 267 to learn how to make your own. Avocado oil mayo can be used in tuna salad, for dipping roasted vegetables such as artichokes, or as a creamy base for salad dressing.

We hope this chapter has been useful for you with regard to learning about foods that are often talked about in keto communities. Like we mentioned earlier, you don't *have* to incorporate these items in your nutrition plan, but some can be very helpful for achieving your keto macronutrient combination. Not to mention, many find these additions to be unique and delicious, providing more variety in your grocery cart and meal plans.

Chapter 16

Popular Nutrition Myths, Busted!

For decades, we have been told to eat particular foods in order to obtain certain vitamins, as well as to achieve specific health and wellness goals. Unfortunately, some of these foods that have been touted as superior sources of the nutrients we need are actually lower quality than what we have been led to believe by extensive marketing efforts. The myths we are about to go over stem from general blanket statements that have little to no credible statistics or research to back them up. Unfortunately, these myths—some of which are primary culprits in the deteriorating health of the general population—have spread throughout society as being legitimate and thus are followed by the masses.

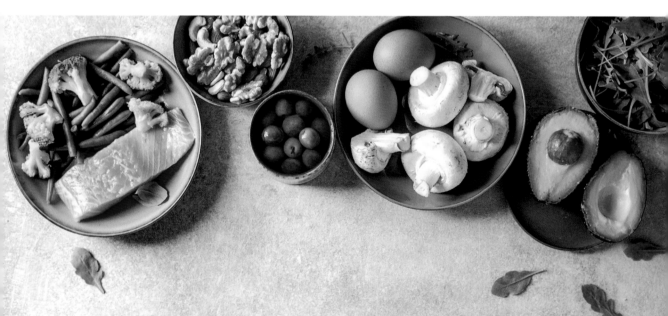

Myth (1) You need whole wheat bread, pasta, and cereal to get your fiber!
The daily recommended fiber amount is 25 grams for women and 38 grams for men. Excellent marketing by the food industry has made people believe that whole wheat bread, whole wheat pasta, and whole-grain cereal are good fiber sources. The truth of the matter is that you can get much more fiber per calorie in other sources of unprocessed, natural foods. Below we compare different food sources of fiber, and illustrate how much one must eat of a particular food to obtain 30 grams of fiber.

Food	Calories Consumed to Reach 30 Grams of Fiber	Carbohydrates Consumed to Reach 30 Grams of Fiber	Sodium Consumed to Reach 30 Grams of Fiber
Whole Wheat Bread	1,350	270g	2,025mg
Multi-Grain Cereal	1,275	275g	2,300mg
Whole Wheat Pasta	1,260	246g	20mg
Avocado	702	36g	30mg
Flax Seed	550	30g	30mg
Strawberries	486	117g	6mg
Broccoli	465	90g	450mg
Kale	396	72g	300mg
Chia Seeds	385	33g	13mg
Raspberries	240	56g	4mg
Artichoke Hearts	195	45g	200mg

In addition to having more fiber per calorie, natural foods such as avocado, flax seeds, strawberries, broccoli, kale, chia seeds, raspberries, and artichokes are unprocessed and contain no artificial additives, but most commercially made breads, pastas, and cereals do. Whole foods are superior when it comes to vitamins and minerals, too. Breads and cereals are fortified with vitamins, which means they do not occur naturally and therefore, they are harder to absorb. The next time you are in a grocery store, look at the ingredient labels of breads, pastas, and cereals—you'll find a plethora of ingredients (such as sugar, high-fructose corn syrup, and preservatives) that are not ideal for weight loss, blood sugar, and overall wellness.

Myth (2) You need several servings of whole wheat bread, pasta, and cereal to get your carbs!

Many nutrition resources recommend as much as 355 grams of carbohydrates per day, most of which come from gluten-containing foods such as whole wheat bread, pasta, and cereal. These types of carbohydrates are high glycemic, which means they turn into a lot of sugar! Overconsumption of sugar is one of the primary causes of type 2 diabetes and the sugar you don't burn off turns to fat, so it is critical to keep sugars and high-glycemic carbohydrates to a minimum. In all actuality, there is absolutely no real nutrition need for carbohydrate consumption to come from breads, pastas, cereals, and crackers as low-glycemic options such as green vegetables, berries, and avocado are unprocessed carbohydrate sources that have an abundance of naturally occurring nutrients and fiber.

Myth (3) Don't eat fish due to environmental toxins!

Yes, there are some fish to limit due to high mercury content such as tilefish, shark, and swordfish. On the other hand, there are many types of fish that are extremely beneficial for macro- and micronutrient compositions. Wild salmon, for example is relatively low in mercury but high in protein and omega-3 fatty acids. As discussed previously, omega-3 fatty acids promote a variety of positive health outcomes such as a lowered risk for heart disease, inflammation, arthritis, and Alzheimer's disease. According to the Natural Resources Defense Council, the following listed sea foods are the lowest in mercury.

Anchovies, butterfish, catfish, clam, crab (domestic), crawfish/crayfish, croaker (Atlantic), flounder, haddock (Atlantic), hake, herring, mullet, oyster, perch, plaice, pollack, salmon (canned or fresh), sardine, scallop, shad (American), shrimp, sole (Pacific), squid (calamari), trout (freshwater), whitefish

* You will see in following chapters, that some 30-day keto plan meals and recipes incorporate canned tuna. If you are one who eats several servings of fish per week and are concerned about mercury intake, we recommend chunk-light tuna since it is three times lower in mercury than solid white albacore.

Myth ④ Drink lots of milk to get your calcium!

Once again, the marketing for milk has been genius—it does a body good, right? Well, maybe not so much. First of all, as mentioned earlier, cow's milk has hormones in it, which help to grow very large cows! Even if you choose the organic brands, the hormones (intended for cows) still remain. Milk is touted for its calcium content and is known for building strong bones but some studies suggest that calcium found in cow's milk has no correlation with strong bones and prevention of fractures.[1] Not to mention, at 12 grams of sugar per cup, it's not the ideal beverage for weight loss and blood sugar levels. For more beneficial sources of calcium, please refer to the table at right.

Food	Serving	Calories	Calcium (mg)	Sugar (g)
Sardines	3.5 ounces	210	351	0
Sesame seeds	¼ cup	206	351	0
Collard greens (cooked)	1 cup	49	300	1
Spinach (cooked)	1 cup	41	245	1
Canned salmon	4 ounces	155	232	0
Fresh wild salmon	6 ounces	300	120	0
Kale (raw)	1 cup	33	101	0
Almonds	23 almonds	162	75	1
Broccoli	1 cup	31	74	1.5
Butternut squash	1 cup	63	67	3

Myth ⑤ Eggs will give you bad cholesterol and put you at risk for heart disease!

Despite eggs being a nutritious whole food, in 1968, the American Heart Association announced that all individuals should eat no more than three eggs per week due to their cholesterol content. Eggs also include invaluable vitamins and minerals, including vitamins B2, B5, B7, B12, and D, as well as omega-3 fats, high-quality protein, choline, iodine, selenium, and zinc. Because eggs contain cholesterol, they have been labeled as an unhealthy food that will contribute to raised LDL (bad) cholesterol and therefore, result in

---

1 D. Feskanich et al., "Milk, dietary calcium, and bone fractures in women: a 12-year prospective study.," NCBI, June 1997, accessed September 11, 2017, ncbi.nlm.nih.gov/pmc/articles/PMC1380936/.

putting one at higher risk for heart disease. In 2015, the restriction of egg intake was eliminated from US dietary guidelines since there is lacking evidence that cholesterol from egg consumption actually causes heart disease. Many mainstream recommendations urge to consume cereal or oatmeal for breakfast due to being "heart healthy" despite the fact that those selections raise blood sugar (while eggs do not), but studies have shown that eating two eggs for breakfast in place of oatmeal reflects no change or increase in biomarkers related to heart disease.[2] In fact, more than fifty years' worth of research has shown that the cholesterol in eggs has very little impact on LDL cholesterol levels, and is not associated with increased cardiovascular disease risk. Moreover, egg intake compensates for an array of common nutritional inadequacies, contributing to overall health and life span.[3]

Myth (6) You need fortified milk, juice, and cereal for vitamin D.

Vitamin D intake is critical for bone and tooth health and support of the nervous and immune system; it also promotes lung and cardiovascular health and may be associated with cancer prevention. Vitamin D is also one of the most common nutritional deficiencies due to the fact that it can be hard to find in foods. Below you will find a list of keto-approved foods that have vitamin D, however, if you are one of the millions who are deficient in the vitamin, you may want to consider responsible sun exposure (around 10 to 15 minutes per day with no sunscreen) or consult with your doctor about supplementing.

Source	International Units (IU) Per Serving
Fish oil	1,000
Sockeye salmon (3 ounces)	447
Canned tuna (3 ounces)	154
Some brands of yogurt (6 ounces)	80
Sardines (2 whole sardines)	46
Beef liver, cooked (3 ounces)*	42
Whole egg (1 large)	41
Swiss cheese (1 ounce)	6

---

2   Missimer, A., D. DiMarco, C. Andersen, A. Murillo, M. Vergara-Jiminez, and M. Fernandez. "Consuming Two Eggs per Day, as Compared to an Oatmeal Breakfast, Decreases Plasma Ghrelin While Maintaining the LDL/HDL Ratio." NCBI. February 01, 2017. Accessed April 27, 2019. ncbi.nlm.nih.gov/pmc/articles/PMC5331520/.

3   McNamara, Donald. "The Fifty Year Rehabilitation of the Egg." NCBI. October 2015. Accessed April 27, 2019. ncbi.nlm.nih.gov/pmc/articles/PMC4632449/.

Myth (7) You need fortified foods to get your folate!

Folate (otherwise known as B9) is famously known due to being imperative during pregnancy to prevent neural tube defects, however, folate is extremely important for the rest of the population, too. Folate is required to produce red and white blood cells in the bone marrow, create DNA and RNA, and convert carbohydrates into energy. Synthetic folic acid (the manufactured form of natural folate) is added to a variety of processed foods such as breads, cereals, and pastas, and one of the primary reasons these blood-sugar-raising foods are touted as being healthy is because they contain fortified nutrients such as folic acid. Unfortunately, 40 percent of the population cannot metabolize synthetic folic acid, so consumption of these products may not help you meet your goal of required folic acid intake. There are, however, a large variety of low-carbohydrate whole foods that boast substantial amounts of naturally occurring folate which is far more bioavailable with higher absorption rates. See below for a chart of folate-rich foods.

Food Source	Serving Size	Folate Per Serving (mcg)
Cooked asparagus	1 cup	262
Cooked okra	1 cup	206
Cooked spinach	1 cup	200
Cooked collard greens	1 cup	177
Turnip greens	1 cup	170
Cooked brussels sprouts	1 cup	160
Raw spinach	1 cup	110
Mustard greens	1 cup	103
Cooked broccoli	1 cup	100
Sunflower seeds	¼ cup	82
Strawberries	8 cedium	80
Cooked cauliflower	1 cup	70
Romaine lettuce	1 cup	65
Avocado	½ cup	55
Flax seeds	2 tablespoons	54
Green beans	1 cup	42

Myth (8) You can get everything you need from vitamins!

Synthetic vitamin intake (as opposed to obtaining naturally occurring vitamins from food) has become a popular, quick fix among the general population. Store-bought multivitamins are synthetic versions of real vitamins—they are made in a lab! Typical food intake and the standard American diet lacks essential vitamins and nutrients, which creates the need for the ever-expanding market of fortified nutrients. If you eat a balanced diet of whole foods, you will get what you need for your health and wellness goals. Standard multivitamins are not easily absorbed and contain things like folic acid and ferrous sulfate—inferior versions of folate and iron that have low absorption rates, as well as side effects.

Myth (9) Stay away from fat!

It is true that many fats should be limited but not all fats are created equally! We tend to overdose on omega-6 fats, which are found in items such as processed foods, vegetable oil, fast food, cookies, chips, and French fries, and then lack the omega-3 fats that are most beneficial for weight loss and heart health. Polyunsaturated omega-3 fats found in foods such as wild salmon, walnuts, flax seeds, seaweed, and grass-fed meats are not only beneficial for weight loss and lowered blood sugar levels, they are also associated with the lowering of blood pressure and risk for heart disease. Besides polyunsaturated fats, monounsaturated fats found in extra-virgin olive oil, avocado, and almonds also assist with weight loss, reduction of the risk of heart disease, and inflammation.

You will receive a lot of advice (good and bad) when it comes to nutrition—hopefully, we have cleared up some confusion for you by dispelling some of these popular myths. Nutrition can be complicated due to the never-ending and conflicting resources that are available in books and on the internet today. As previously mentioned, many aspects of nutrition science have come from funded studies by special interest groups, so it is always best to scratch beneath the surface of some popular myths and recommendations and do your own research.

Chapter 17

Welcome to "Almost Keto"—
Your Long-Term Plan

As you may know, there are several forms of the ketogenic diet. In fact, there are several forms of all nutrition plans as different variations work for different people. Here are descriptions of six popular keto trends, all of which have different rules and guidelines. Spoiler alert—none of these will be your wean-off plan!

- **Standard Ketogenic Diet:** Presumably the most popular form of keto, it typically calls for 75 percent fat, 20 percent protein, and only 5 percent carbohydrates. Extremely low in carbohydrates (calling for less than 50 grams of carbohydrates per day), and high in fat, while moderate in protein.
- **"Dirty" Keto Diet:** One of the newer and fairly common keto trends, "dirty keto" follows the same macronutrient protocol (75 percent fat, 20 percent protein, and 5 percent carbohydrates) but it doesn't matter what foods those macros come from. Technically, one can eat unlimited amounts of bun-less fast food burgers, pork rinds, and bacon as long as those macros are in alignment.
- **"Lazy" Keto Diet:** This version of keto doesn't call for tracking the amounts of protein and fat one consumes, however, the "lazy keto" dieter does track carbohydrates with the intention of remaining as low as under 20 grams per day.
- **Cyclical Ketogenic Diet:** This form of keto involves short periods of higher-carbohydrate intake, such as six standard ketogenic days followed by one high-carbohydrate day, also known as a "refeed" day. The refeed day consists of roughly 150 grams of carbohydrates.
- **Targeted Ketogenic Diet:** Specifically for high-intensity athletes and body builders, this version of keto is very similar to the Standard Ketogenic Diet, however, it focuses on adding in the daily allotted carbohydrates around workout times for added energy.

- **High-Protein Ketogenic Diet:** Similar to the Standard Ketogenic Diet, it includes a slightly lower amount of fat, with more protein, and the same amount of carbohydrates. The ratio is often 60 percent fat, 35 percent protein, and 5 percent carbohydrates.

The wean-off plan we have formulated for you is called *almost keto,* and it employs all of the foods you have been working with in this book. However, the macronutrient composition will be different—many feel it's easier, healthier, and more sustainable for the long-term. In fact, you'll be cutting your fat intake substantially and the best news (for some) is that you will have more room for low-glycemic carbohydrates by way of green vegetables and low-sugar fruits. And you may be pleasantly surprised to see a few new foods that were too high in carbohydrates to be used during your 30-day plan, but can be eaten in moderation now. Your food plan will still be low in carbohydrates and sugar, compared to the standard American diet, so you will still see your results progress and be maintained. Here is your simple four-step guide to getting started on your *almost keto* maintenance plan.

Step (1) Understand your macronutrients.

The newly adjusted *almost keto* guidelines for fat, protein, and carbohydrates will be different than the standard keto protocol. The suggested guideline (give or take) for your new dietary intake is 45 percent fat, 30 percent protein, and 25 percent carbohydrates.

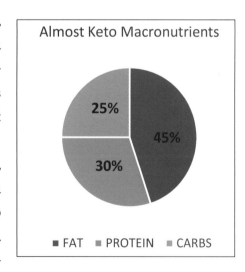

Almost Keto Macronutrients

25%

45%

30%

■ FAT ■ PROTEIN ■ CARBS

To be clear, to consume 45 percent fat in your diet, it means to get 45 percent of all of your calories from fat. For example, if you eat 2,000 calories per day, 900 of your total calories must come from fat sources. Thirty percent of your calories will come from protein, so 600 calories will be from protein sources. Twenty-five percent of your calories will come from carbohydrates since 500 calories is 25 percent of your 2,000 calories. To take the guesswork out, below is a table that shows how many grams of fat, protein, and carbohydrates you need from a variety of daily caloric intake requirements, starting with 1,200 per day and ending with 3,500 per day. Although the average number of calories to consume is 2,000 per day, it will be different for each individual since required calories are determined by current weight, goal weight, gender, age, and activity level. Free calorie calculators can be accessed online so you can determine what is best for you and your goals.

Keep in mind, the following chart is a general guideline to give you an idea of the amounts of calories and macronutrients to consume to achieve certain weight goals. Does this mean you need to religiously adhere to calorie, fat, protein, and carbohydrate counting? Absolutely not! By sticking to the green and orange foods list found later in this chapter, your macronutrients will naturally fall into place.

Total Calories	Fat Calories	Grams of Fat	Protein Calories	Grams of Protein	Carbohydrate Calories	Grams of Carbohydrates	Daily Total
1,200	540	60	360	90	300	75	1,200 calories 60 grams of fat 90 grams of protein 75 grams of carbs
1,500	675	75	450	112	375	94	1,500 calories 75 grams of fat 112 grams of protein 94 grams of carbs
2,000	900	100	600	150	500	125	2,000 calories 100 grams of fat 150 grams of protein 125 grams of carbs
2,500	1,125	125	750	187	625	156	2,500 calories 125 grams of fat 187 grams of protein 156 grams of carbs
3,000	1 350	150	900	225	750	187	3,000 calories 150 grams of fat 225 grams of protein 187 grams of carbs
3,500	1,575	175	1050	262	875	219	3,500 calories 175 grams of fat 262 grams of protein 219 grams of carbs

* Calorie to gram conversions are based on nine calories per gram of fat, four calories per gram of protein, and four calories per gram of carbohydrate.

Since you're already familiar with the keto lifestyle, you may be wondering if the above carbohydrate counts are for total carbohydrates or "net carbohydrates." The *almost keto* way of counting carbohydrates is simply going by total carbs on the nutrition label. Standard keto protocols suggest subtracting grams of fiber and sugar alcohols from total carbohydrates to obtain the figure of "net carbohydrates," however, *almost keto* is already a bit higher in carbs and for ease of less calculation, we will just go by regular carbohydrate numbers.

Step ② Focus on higher-quality fats.

As with standard keto, *almost keto* will still require you to focus on some fats but they will not be as large of a proportion of your nutrition plan as you are not aiming to "get into ketosis" to reach your goals. With *almost keto,* we still ask you to choose fats mindfully, opting for the better versions and avoiding regular use of foods such as bacon, hot dogs, deli meats, pork rinds, and low-carb processed and fast foods. Keep choosing healthy fats that are monounsaturated such as extra-virgin olive oil, as well as polyunsaturated fats that have essential omega-3 fatty acids. Keep in mind, quality is more important than quantity, so if forgoing

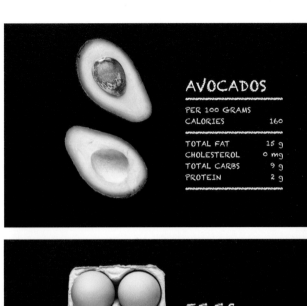

AVOCADOS

PER 100 GRAMS

CALORIES	160

TOTAL FAT	15 g
CHOLESTEROL	0 mg
TOTAL CARBS	9 g
PROTEIN	2 g

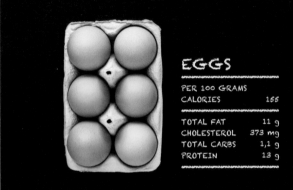

EGGS

PER 100 GRAMS

CALORIES	155

TOTAL FAT	11 g
CHOLESTEROL	373 mg
TOTAL CARBS	1,1 g
PROTEIN	13 g

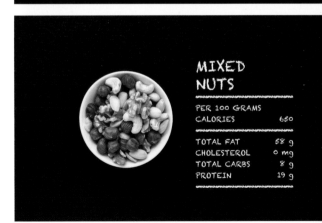

MIXED NUTS

PER 100 GRAMS

CALORIES	650

TOTAL FAT	58 g
CHOLESTEROL	0 mg
TOTAL CARBS	8 g
PROTEIN	19 g

an unhealthy fat (such as vegetable oil) means that you won't quite hit your 45 percent fat quota, that is perfectly fine. Here is a snapshot of some of our favorite fat recommendations, however, you can still refer back to chapter 4 for your complete list of approved fats.

Step ③ Get your grocery list.

Now that you know how many calories and grams of fat, protein, and carbohydrates you should be consuming, it's time to talk about food. The foods that will make up these *almost keto* percentages are keto-approved, meaning they are in alignment with all standard keto guildelines as they are low in carbohydrates and sugar, however, they are mostly cleaner keto foods. Foods found in the green list can be eaten as much as you like and in any combination to obtain your *almost keto* percentages of macronutrients of 45 percent fat, 30 percent protein, and 25 percent carbohydrates. Foods found in the orange list should be limited or consumed in moderation due to being higher in carbohydrates and sugar or having additives that are not ideal for overall well-being.

Below you will find your Green Keto Foods list. The foods found in this category are the cleanest and most effective for your *almost keto* regimen.

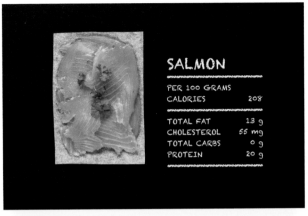

SALMON

PER 100 GRAMS
CALORIES   208

TOTAL FAT   13 g
CHOLESTEROL   55 mg
TOTAL CARBS   0 g
PROTEIN   20 g

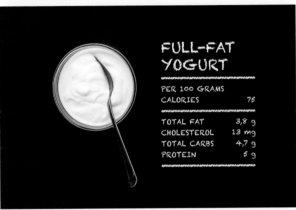

FULL-FAT YOGURT

PER 100 GRAMS
CALORIES   75

TOTAL FAT   3,8 g
CHOLESTEROL   13 mg
TOTAL CARBS   4,7 g
PROTEIN   5 g

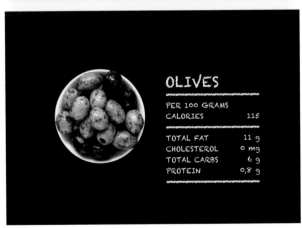

OLIVES

PER 100 GRAMS
CALORIES   115

TOTAL FAT   11 g
CHOLESTEROL   0 mg
TOTAL CARBS   6 g
PROTEIN   0,8 g

Green Keto Foods

Fatty Foods and Condiments	Animal and Vegan Proteins	Low-Sugar Vegetables	Low-Sugar Fruits	Cooking Extras
Avocado	Amaranth	Artichoke hearts	Avocado	Almond milk
Avocado oil	Artichokes	Arugula	Bell pepper	Apple cider vinegar
Chia seeds	Asparagus	Asparagus	Blackberries	Avocado oil
Chicken (skin on)	Bison	Aubergines	Blueberries	Basil
Coconut milk	Broccoli	Bok choy	Lemon	Black pepper
Coconut oil	Chia seeds	Broccoli	Lime	Cilantro
Dark chocolate (at least 70 percent)	Chicken	Brussels sprouts	Olives	Cinnamon
Eggs	Clams	Cabbage	Raspberries	Coconut aminos
Extra-virgin olive oil	Cod	Cauliflower	Strawberries	Coconut milk
Flax seeds	Crab	Celery	Tomato	Coconut oil
Grass-fed/organic beef	Eggs	Collard greens		Extra-virgin olive oil
Greek yogurt	Grass-fed beef	Eggplant		Flax seed oil
Herring	Halibut	Green beans		Garlic
Krill oil (Supplement)	Hemp seeds	Kale		Ginger
Lamb	Lamb	Kimchi		Nutritional yeast
Macadamia nuts	Mackerel	Leeks		Oregano
Macadamia oil	Mussels	Mushrooms		Paleo mayo
Mackerel	Natto	Peppers		Parsley
MCT oil	Octopus	Pickles		Rosemary
Olives	Oysters	Radishes		Sage
Oysters	Pork	Romaine lettuce		Sea salt
Paleo mayo	Rockfish	Sauerkraut		Soy aminos
Pecans	Salmon (fresh or canned)	Spinach		Tahini
Pine nuts	Scallops			Tamari
Pork chop	Shrimp			Tarragon
Pumpkin seeds	Sole			Thyme
Seaweed	Spinach			Turmeric
Sunflower butter	Spirulina			
Sunflower seeds	Squid			
Tahini	Tempeh			
Tuna	Tuna (fresh or canned)			
Walnuts	Turkey			
Wild salmon (fresh or canned)	Venison			
Wild salmon oil (supplement)	Walnuts			

You probably noticed that some of the traditional keto staples are missing—items such as bacon, butter, cheese, and pork rinds. Though these items are high in fat and meet the macronutrient guidelines for the keto protocol, there are a variety of reasons (including but not limited to carcinogens, hormones found in dairy, excessive omega-6 fatty acids, as well as additives and preservatives) why the *almost keto* protocol does not endorse unlimited use of these products. The following Orange Keto Foods List includes many of these foods for your convenience, however, we urge *limited to moderate consumption* at most. In addition, you will notice a few items found on the Orange List that are not part of the Standard Keto Diet as the *almost keto* regimen has a little more leniency for carbohydrate consumption. They do hold an optional place in the *almost keto* regimen for the sake of particular macro- and micronutrients, and for wider nutrition plan variety, especially for those who may enjoy more plant-based foods.

Orange Keto Foods

Fatty Foods	Animal and Vegan Proteins	Higher-Sugar Fruits and Vegetables
Almond butter	Almond butter	Apple
Bacon	Bacon	Apricot
Butter	Beans	Banana
Cashew butter	Deli meats	Cantaloupe
Cashews	Hard cheese	Carrots
Cheese	Lentils	Cherries
Chestnuts	Peanut butter	Grapefruit
Cottage cheese	Peas	Grapes
Cream	Pork rinds	Honeydew melon
Deli meats	Quinoa	Kiwi
Ghee	Soft cheese	Nectarines
Peanut butter		Oranges
Pork rinds		Peaches
		Pears
		Pineapple
		Plums
		Pomegranate
		Watermelon
		Winter squash

Step (4) Know what you shouldn't be eating.

Just as in your 30-day plan, *almost-keto-approved* foods help you lose weight and improve blood sugar levels because they are low in carbohydrates and low in sugar. Some of these red-listed foods may be touted as "healthy" or "weight-loss-friendly" in some circles, however, the sugar and carbohydrate content will negate your efforts.

Any foods that are moderate to high in either carbohydrates or sugar should be eliminated or severely limited to see results.

You may be wondering if you need to purchase all of the green list items in order to start your *almost keto* regimen, and the answer is no! The wide variety of foods found in the green list gives you flexibility with regard to your food lifestyle, possible allergies, and aversions. Feel free to pick and choose the green groceries you prefer the most. As mentioned previously, you are not required to count calories and macronutrients as sticking to the *almost keto* green list, as well as the *almost keto* Perfect 10 Foods (found back in chapter 4) will help to ensure you are consuming proper amounts of fat, protein, and carbohydrates.

Bagels
Cake
Candy
Cereal
Commercial granola bars
Cookies
Crackers
Croissants
Donuts
Fast food and processed foods (even low-carb versions)
Fruit juice
Ice cream
Muffins
Other sugary beverages
Pita bread
Pita chips
Pizza crust
Potato chips
Potatoes
Rice
Soda
Tortillas
White or whole wheat bread
White or whole wheat flour
White or whole wheat pasta

Chapter 18

30-Day Keto Breakfast Recipes

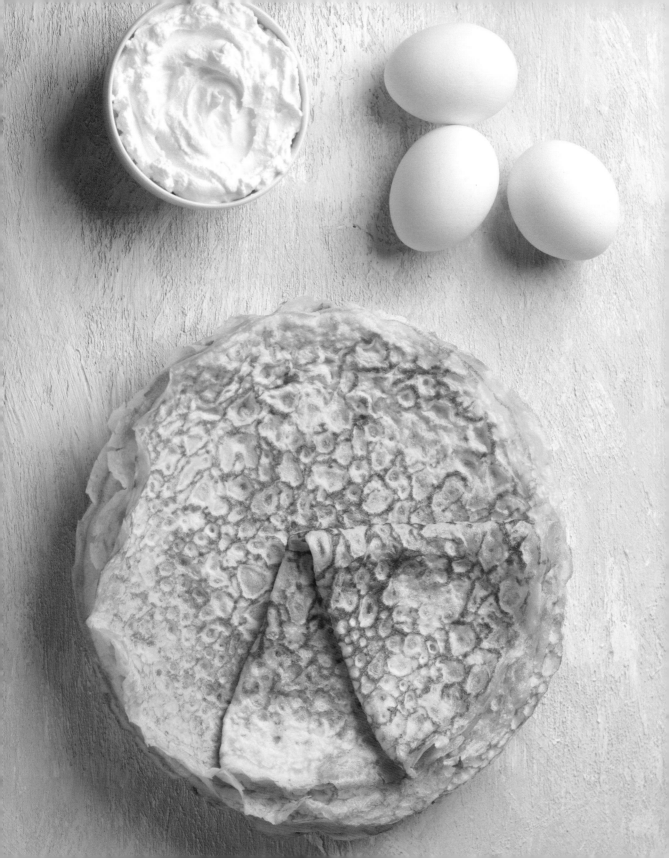

Keto Pancakes

These crepe-like pancakes are a favorite in the keto community and they are very low in carbohydrates and sugar. Closer to a true French crepe, this variation is not as fluffy as the pancake recipe found on page 88. You can top them with berries, nut butters, bacon crumbles, and butter, or salmon and crème fraîche, or they can be filled with cheese, onions, bell peppers, and mushrooms, folded over, and eaten like a stuffed savory crepe.

Serves 2

Ingredients:

½ cup cream cheese, softened
3 large eggs
3 tablespoons almond flour
Pinch of salt (optional)
Pinch of cinnamon (optional)
Butter for cooking

Steps:

1. Place all ingredients except butter in a blender and blend for 1 minutes.

2. Using butter, spoon batter into a hot pan and cook for 1 minute on each side.

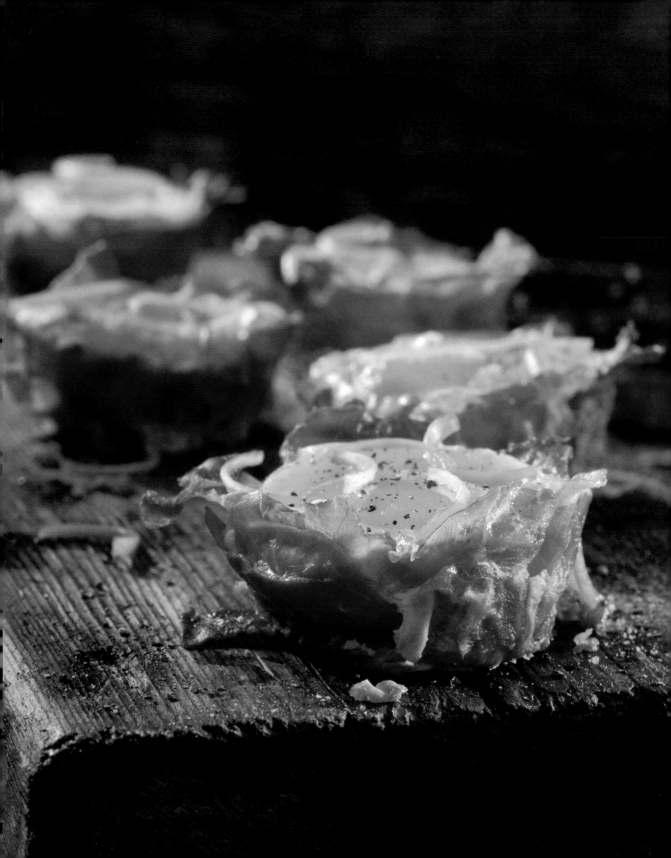

Prosciutto Egg Cups

These egg cups can be made ahead of time and taken on the go for a delicious and keto-friendly breakfast. For an impressive breakfast or brunch, multiply these ingredients by six and fill a 12-muffin tin, and pair with mixed greens and sparkling mineral water.

Serves 1 (2 egg cups)

Ingredients:

2 eggs
1 scallion, thinly sliced
1 tablespoon unsweetened full-fat coconut milk
Pepper, to taste
1 teaspoon coconut oil
2 prosciutto slices, folded in half

Steps:

1. Preheat oven to 350°F.

2. In a small bowl, beat the eggs and combine with scallion.

3. Mix in the coconut milk and add freshly ground pepper, to taste.

4. Using the coconut oil, grease 2 muffin tin spaces, and line each cup with 1 folded prosciutto slice.

5. Using the egg mixture, fill each cup until ⅔ full.

6. Bake for 30 minutes, until eggs are cooked through.

Avocado-Kale Egg Skillet

This egg dish is filled with fresh produce for the healthiest carbohydrates, and a delicious combination of flavors. Chilled sliced tomatoes drizzled with extra-virgin olive oil and sea salt are the perfect low-sugar compliment.

Serves 1

Ingredients:

Handful fresh kale, stemmed and sliced
1 tablespoon avocado oil, divided
½ cup sliced mushrooms
½ avocado, sliced
2 eggs
Salt and pepper, to taste

Steps:

1. In a small bowl, massage the kale with half of the avocado oil. Set aside to let it tenderize.

2. In a medium skillet over medium heat, heat the other half of the oil.

3. Add the mushrooms to the pan and sauté for 2 minutes.

4. Place the kale on top of the mushrooms, then place the slices of avocado on top of the kale.

5. Create 2 wells for the eggs, and crack 1 egg into each well. Season the skillet with salt and pepper, to taste.

6. Cover the skillet and cook until the eggs have set, around 5 minutes.

7. Serve hot.

Eggs in a Hole

A low-carbohydrate take on the old classic, these eggs are encased in bell-pepper instead of high-glycemic bread. The bell peppers have a wonderful contrasting taste and texture to the eggs, and this dish pairs nicely with either tomatoes or fresh berries.

Serves 1

Ingredients:

1 teaspoon extra-virgin olive oil
2½-inch sliced bell pepper rings
2 eggs
Salt and pepper, to taste

Steps:

1. In a medium skillet, heat extra-virgin olive oil over medium heat. Add bell pepper rings and sauté on one side for 2 minutes and then flip over.

2. Crack the eggs into each of the bell pepper rings and reduce heat to low. Cook the eggs through, about 10 minutes.

3. Add salt and pepper to taste, and serve warm, paired with tomatoes or berries.

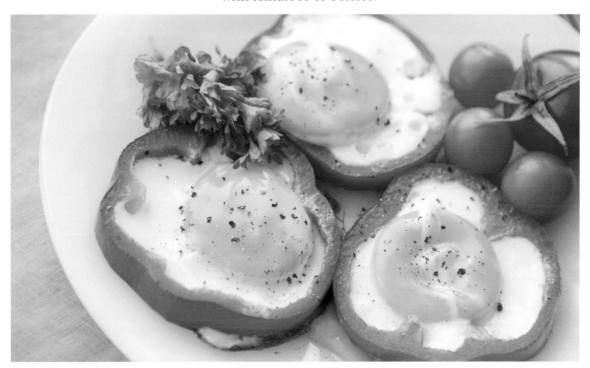

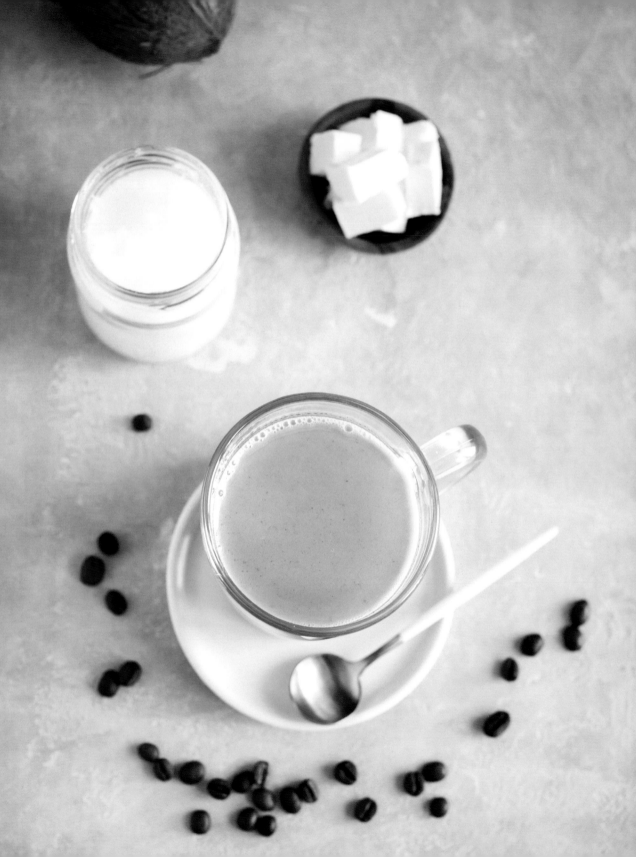

Keto Coffee

Keto coffee is calorie dense and will give you what you need for energy in the morning, even if you don't have time to prepare a traditional breakfast. If you're feeling like something more, pair with 2 eggs and sliced tomatoes, but this filling coffee can stand on its own!

Serves 1

Ingredients:

8 ounces brewed, hot coffee
½ cup unsweetened almond milk or unsweetened coconut milk, heated
1 tablespoon butter or ghee
1 tablespoon MCT oil

Steps:

1. Add all ingredients in blender, and blend for 15 seconds until frothy.

Cream Cheese and Lox Sliders

Your cream cheese and lox sliders can be made with just a few ingredients. For a light and refreshing twist, opt for sliced cucumber in place of the biscuits.

Serves 2 (4 sliders)

Ingredients:

1 batch 5-Minute Coffee Cup Biscuits (page 189)
3 ounces whipped cream cheese
3 ounces wild lox, chopped
Fresh dill, for garnish
Capers, for garnish
Freshly squeezed lemon, to taste

Steps:

1. Spread equal amounts of cream cheese on each of the 4 biscuits.

2. Top each cream cheese biscuit with equal amounts of chopped lox.

3. Garnish each biscuit with fresh dill and capers, and top with a sprinkle of lemon juice.

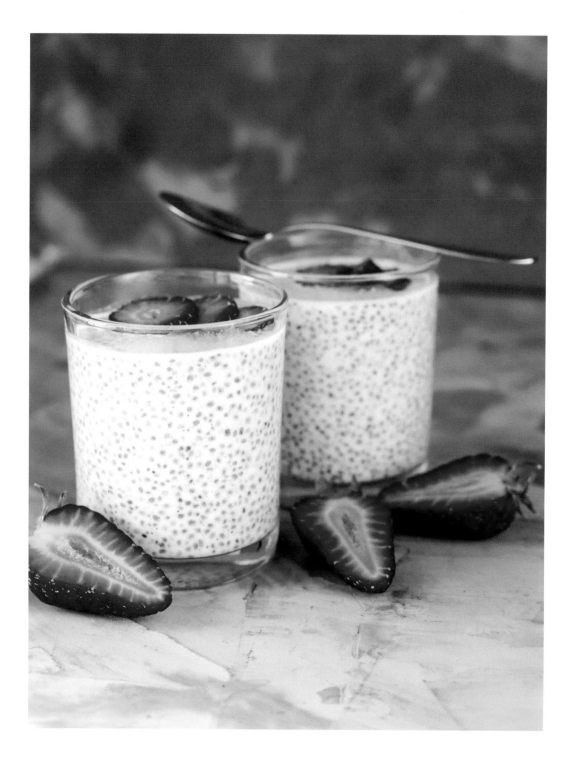

Easy Chia Seed Breakfast Pudding

This breakfast pudding only takes minutes to prepare and refrigerate overnight if you're looking for a quick and unique breakfast idea. If you're looking for added protein and like the combination of sweet and savory, simply pair with a slice or two of bacon.

Serves 1

Ingredients:

½ cup unsweetened coconut milk
1½ tablespoons chia seeds
½ teaspoon vanilla extract
Fresh berries (optional)

Steps:

1. Combine coconut milk, chia seeds, and vanilla in small bowl or jar.

2. Cover and refrigerate for at least 2 hours, or overnight.

3. Top with your favorite berries (optional).

Bacon and Egg Breakfast Caesar Salad

This dish takes the classic Caesar salad and gives it a breakfast twist, and it's a unique way to add some greens into your day from the start. To make this salad ahead of time, simply hard-boil the eggs (instead of frying or poaching) and dice. This version keeps well overnight and can be taken on the go.

Serves 1

Ingredients:

2 strips of bacon
1 teaspoon oil
2 eggs
2 cups chopped romaine lettuce
Caesar dressing, to taste (page 271)

Steps:

1. Pan-cook the bacon over medium-low heat, turning over periodically until cooked through, about 10 minutes.

2. While the bacon is cooking, using oil, pan-cook the eggs over medium-low heat for 3 minutes. Reduce heat to low and cover until cooked through, around 5 additional minutes.

3. While the eggs and bacon are cooking, chop the lettuce and place in a medium bowl.

4. Chop the bacon strips and add to the lettuce. Toss in the Caesar dressing.

5. Add the eggs on top of your salad and serve.

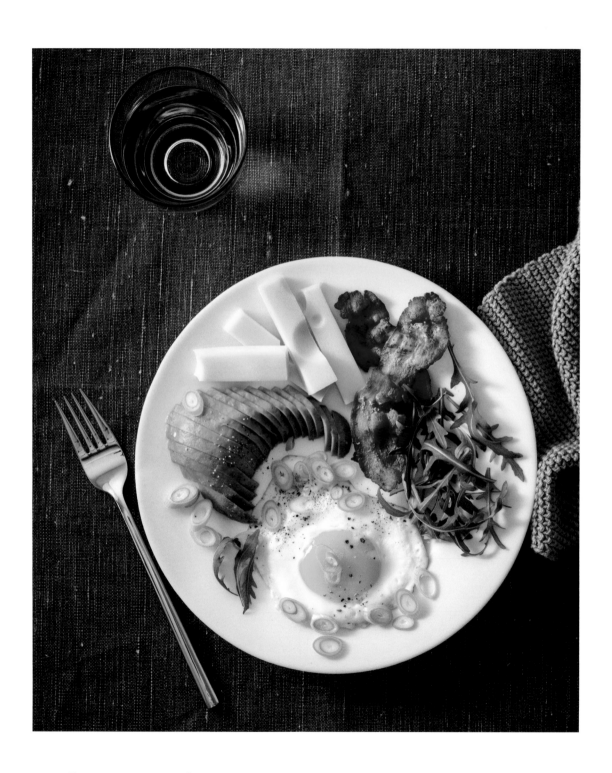

Bacon and Egg Platter

This dish is a bit more delectable and varied compared to the regular bacon and eggs breakfast. If you're cooking for a group, simply multiply the recipe and be sure to impress your friends if you're hosting a keto-friendly Sunday brunch. Garnishing with fresh arugula adds more vitamins and minerals, and complements the avocado.

Serves 1

Ingredients:

2 pieces bacon
1 ounce cheese, sliced
½ avocado, sliced
Handful arugula
1 egg

Steps:

1. Pan-cook bacon over medium-low heat, turning over every 2 minutes, until cooked through, about 10 minutes. While the bacon is cooking, plate the cheese, avocado, and arugula.

2. Plate the bacon and carefully crack the egg into the hot bacon grease and cook through, about 5 minutes.

5-Minute Coffee Cup Biscuits

These fluffy biscuits are made from keto-approved ingredients and only take a few minutes to make. Our favorite way to enjoys these is topped with butter or ghee, paired with fresh strawberries, or topped with cream cheese and lox.

Serves 2 (4 biscuits)

Ingredients:

1 large egg
3 tablespoons almond flour
1 tablespoon coconut flour
1 tablespoon soft butter
1 tablespoon avocado oil
¼ teaspoon baking powder
Pinch of salt

Steps:

1. Using a fork, thoroughly combine all ingredients in a microwave-safe mug until the mixture is smooth. Using the back of a spoon, smooth out the top into an even surface.

2. Microwave for 1 minute (based on your microwave, you may have to slightly alter the time and experiment with high versus medium-high temperatures).

3. Using a potholder or thick cloth, remove the hot mug from the microwave. Cover with a plate and turn upside down, allowing the biscuit to slide out of the coffee cup. Slice into 4 even pieces.

4. Serve with butter or ghee, and sliced strawberries.

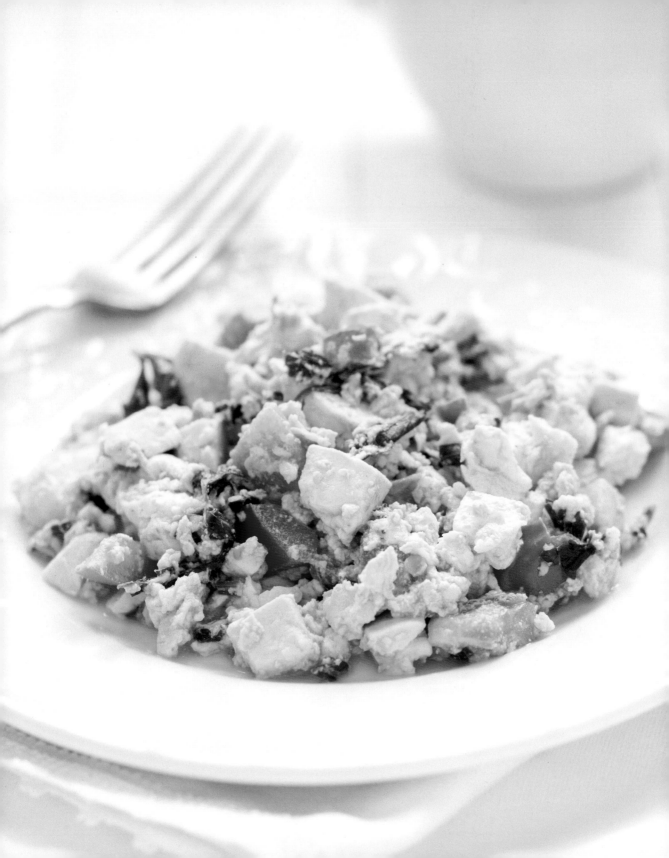

Cheesy Tofu Scramble

This tofu scramble topped with nutritional yeast is reminiscent of a cheesy egg scramble, and it's made with an alternative for those who do not consume eggs. Pair this dish with your favorite berries and you'll have an egg-free breakfast that is packed with protein, healthy fats, fiber, and antioxidants.

Serves 4

Ingredients:

16 ounces organic tofu
1 tablespoon avocado oil
1 bell pepper, sliced
½ onion, diced
1 cup raw spinach
½ teaspoon salt
½ teaspoon black pepper
½ teaspoon onion powder
½ teaspoon garlic powder
¼ teaspoon turmeric
1 tablespoon lemon juice
1 tablespoon nutritional
    yeast

Steps:

1. Drain tofu from its container, wrap in a paper towel, and place on a plate. Rest a heavy plate on top of the wrapped tofu and microwave for 4 minutes.

2. Unwrap the tofu and cut into cubes. Place the tofu cubes in a medium bowl and mash with a fork.

3. Heat the avocado oil in a medium pan over medium heat. Add the bell pepper and onion and cook until slightly tender.

4. Add the spinach to the pan and cook for 3 minutes until spinach as wilted.

5. Add the tofu and cook on medium heat until most of the water has evaporated.

6. Add the salt, pepper, onion powder, garlic powder, and turmeric and thoroughly combine so that all seasonings are evenly distributed.

7. Add the lemon juice and stir well.

8. Remove from heat, plate, and top with nutritional yeast.

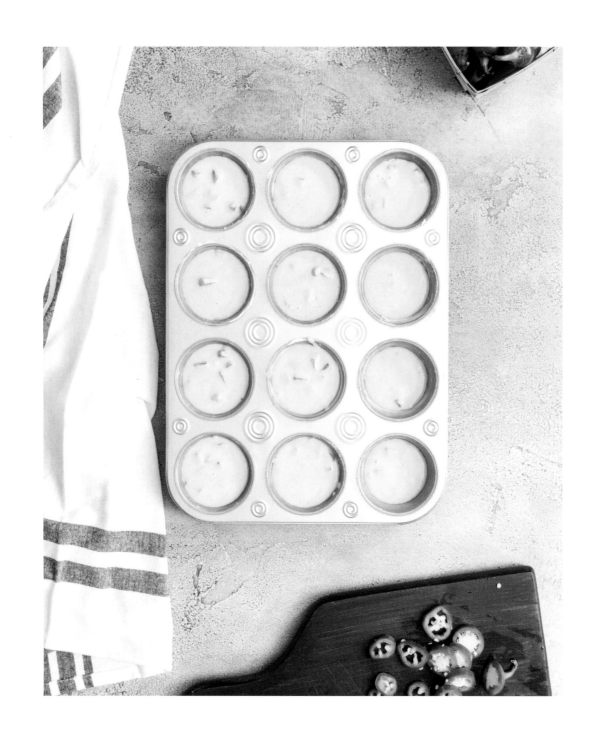

Jalapeño Cream Cheese Muffins

This recipe is great for when you're craving a moist and decadent baked good while adhering to your keto macros. Also, if spicy jalapeño peppers aren't your thing, just replace them with blueberries or strawberries for a sweeter muffin.

Serves 3 (makes 6 muffins)

Ingredients:

4 tablespoons melted butter or ghee, plus more for the muffin tin

1 cup almond flour

¾ tablespoon baking powder

2 ounces cream cheese

2 tablespoons heavy whipping cream

2 large eggs, beaten

Handful shredded cheese

1 jalapeño pepper, diced

Steps:

1. Preheat the oven to 400°F. Using butter or ghee, coat six cups of a muffin tin.

2. In a small bowl, combine the almond flour and baking powder.

3. In a medium bowl, first thoroughly combine the cream cheese and whipping cream until smooth. Then add the eggs, shredded cheese, 4 tablespoons of melted butter, and jalapeño, and thoroughly combine.

4. Add the flour mixture to the egg mixture, and beat with a hand mixer until thoroughly mixed.

5. Pour the batter into the prepared muffin cups.

6. Bake until golden brown on top, about 12 minutes.

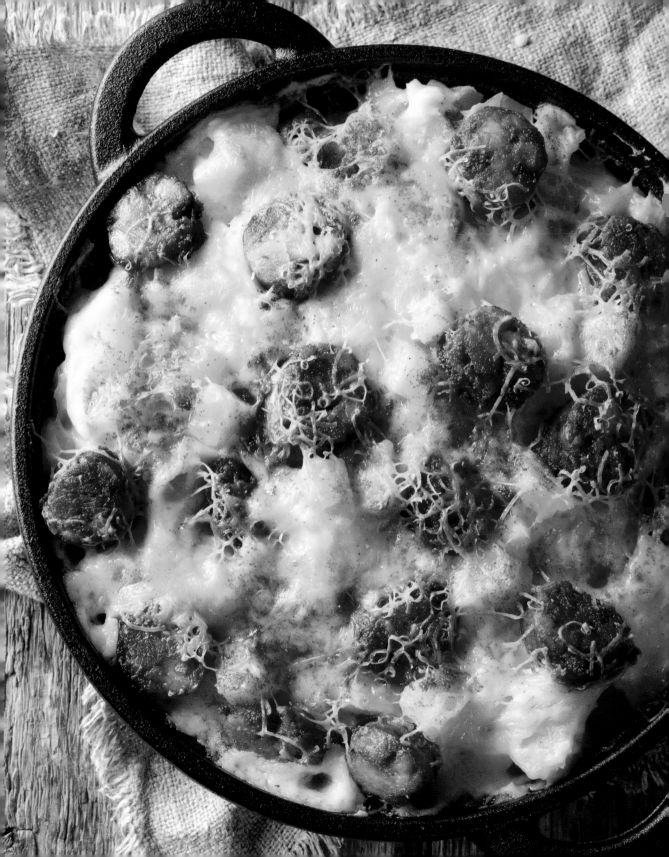

Cheesy Egg and Sausage Bake

This breakfast casserole dish is delicious, not to mention kid-friendly. If you're busy in the mornings, you can prepare, cook, slice, and refrigerate ahead of time. Also, this recipe is tasty on its own, but feel free to experiment with fresh produce additions such as bell pepper, spinach, and mushrooms.

Serves 6

Ingredients:

Avocado oil or nonstick cooking spray for baking dish

1 tablespoon butter or ghee

⅓ cup chopped sweet onions

1 pound breakfast sausage

8 large eggs

⅓ cup heavy whipping cream

1 clove garlic, minced

1 teaspoon salt

Black pepper, to taste

1 cup shredded cheddar cheese

Sour cream, for garnish (optional)

Chopped chives, for garnish (optional)

Steps:

1. Preheat the oven to 350°F. Lightly coat an 8-inch baking dish with avocado oil or non-stick cooking spray.

2. Using butter, sauté the onions over medium heat in a large skillet until soft, 3 to 4 minutes.

3. Add the sausage and cook through, around 5 to 6 minutes. Drain and set aside.

4. In a large bowl, whisk the eggs, cream, garlic, salt, and pepper.

5. Evenly spread the cooked sausage and onion mixture on the bottom of the baking dish and top with an even layer of cheese.

6. Pour the egg mixture over the cheese and bake for 35 minutes until the eggs are set and the top is a light golden brown.

7. Plate and garnish with sour cream and chives (optional).

Grain-Free Breakfast Granola

If you're looking for a cereal replacement that is devoid of grains and filled with protein and healthy fat, grain-free breakfast granola can be topped with your choice of nondairy milk or cream and berries. You'll have enough left over from this recipe to use the granola as a yogurt topping for another breakfast.

Serves 3 (½ cup per serving)

Ingredients:

½ cup raw macadamia nuts

½ cup raw walnuts

¼ cup cacao nibs

2 tablespoons unsweetened coconut flakes

1 teaspoon vanilla extract

1 teaspoon ground cinnamon

¼ teaspoon salt

2 tablespoons coconut oil, melted

Steps:

1. Preheat the oven to 325°F, and line a baking sheet with parchment paper.

2. Using a food processor or knife, finely chop the macadamia nuts and walnuts into small pieces. Combine with cacao nibs, coconut, vanilla, cinnamon, and salt in a medium bowl. Add the coconut oil and mix well.

3. Spread the granola onto the parchment-lined baking sheet and spread evenly into one layer. Bake for 15 minutes or until the granola is toasted at the bottom and fragrant. Keep a close watch and stir frequently as it may burn.

4. Let the granola cool and serve with your favorite nondairy milk.

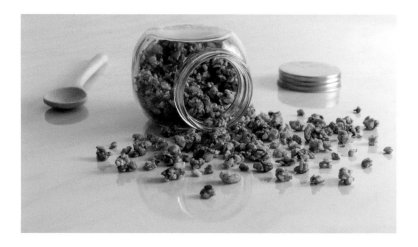

Chapter 19

30-Day Keto Lunch Recipes

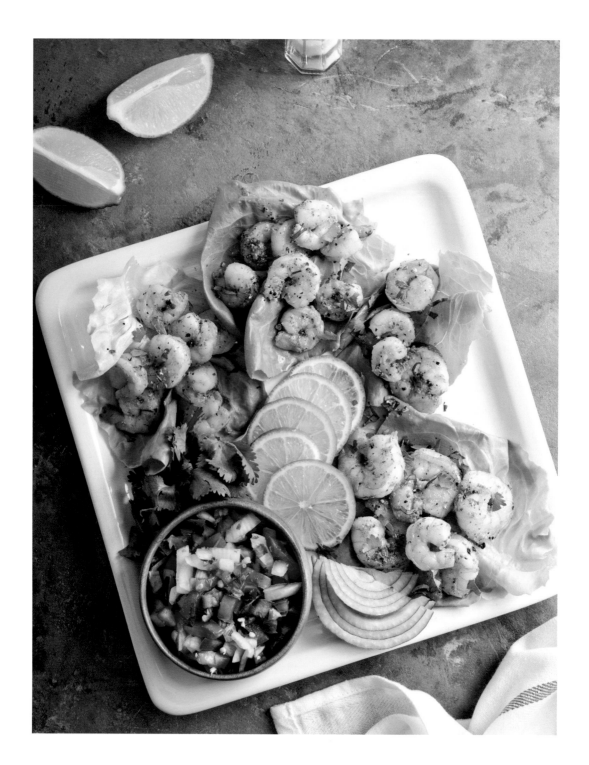

Citrus Shrimp Lettuce Wrap Tacos

You won't miss the tortilla with these bright flavorful shrimp lettuce tacos! This low-carbohydrate dish is filled with all the flavors found in your favorite Mexican dish. You can dress these tacos up with your favorite additions such as salsa, cilantro, and avocado.

Serves 2

Ingredients:

2 tablespoons avocado oil
1 teaspoon ground cumin
½ teaspoon garlic powder
½ teaspoon chili powder
½ teaspoon onion powder
1 teaspoon dried oregano
½ teaspoon paprika
Salt and pepper, to taste
¾ pound medium shrimp
8–10 butter lettuce leaves
½ cup salsa or pico de gallo
Handful cilantro, roughly
    chopped
2 whole limes, halved

Steps:

1. Heat avocado oil in medium-sized pan over medium heat.

2. Add all seasonings to the raw shrimp and toss thoroughly before placing in pan.

3. Cook shrimp for two minutes on the first side, then flip and cook for 3 additional minutes or until shrimp is opaque and cooked through. Remove from heat and set aside.

4. Arrange the butter lettuce leaves on a plate or platter and divide the shrimp evenly into each leaf.

5. Top with salsa or pico de gallo and cilantro, and a generous amount of freshly squeezed lime.

10-Minute No-Bake Chicken Cauliflower Cheese Casserole

If you're in a rush, this no-bake (and no-stove) casserole is a delicious combination of chicken, cauliflower, and cheese. To batch-cook, simply triple the recipe and refrigerate for up to 1 week or freeze for up to 3 months. Pair with grilled asparagus or a small side salad.

Serves 4

Ingredients:

1 pound cauliflower rice

1½ tablespoons water

4 ounces sour cream

1 cup cheddar cheese, shredded

1 pound rotisserie chicken meat (already cooked)

3 tablespoons chives

4 tablespoons butter

1 cup Parmesan cheese

2 teaspoons garlic salt

Salt and pepper, to taste

Steps:

1. Place the cauliflower in a microwave-safe dish with the water. Cover with a piece of plastic wrap, leaving a small gap to let air release.

2. Microwave on high heat for 3 minutes or until tender.

3. Drain excess water from cauliflower and place in a large microwave-safe bowl; mix in all other ingredients.

4. Microwave again on high for 90 seconds and mix again. Serve and enjoy!

Cauliflower Nachos

This cauliflower nacho rendition will give you all of the flavor of traditional nachos while cutting the carbohydrates. Not to mention, the cruciferous vegetable is packed with nutrition, so not only are you not cheating, you're actually getting a delicious meal that is packed with micronutrients.

Serves 4

Ingredients:

1 large head cauliflower
¼ cup avocado oil
1 teaspoon taco seasoning
1 pound ground beef
Salt and pepper, to taste
⅓ cup diced red onion
¾ cup diced tomatoes
1 cup shredded cheddar cheese
1 medium avocado, diced
Sour cream, to taste
Cilantro, to taste
Salsa, to taste

Steps:

1. Preheat oven to 425°F.

2. Cut the cauliflower into florets, and slice the florets into thin "chips."

3. Hand toss the cauliflower chips with the avocado oil and taco seasoning until all is evenly coated. Use more avocado oil if needed to coat all pieces.

4. Put the cauliflower onto the baking sheet in a single layer and roast until edges are browned, about 20 minutes.

5. While the chips are roasting, pan cook the ground beef over medium heat, until cooked through. Break into crumbles as you're cooking, and season with salt and pepper as needed.

6. When the cauliflower is done roasting, flip the pieces over. Top with crumbled ground beef, red onion, tomatoes, and cheddar cheese. Return to the oven until cheese is melted, about 5 minutes.

7. Garnish with avocado, sour cream, cilantro, and salsa, to taste.

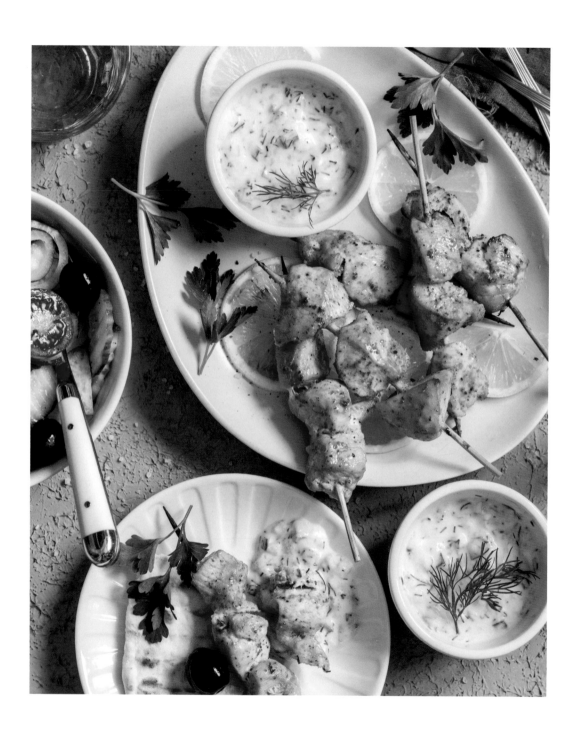

Keto Greek Platter

This hearty Greek platter includes a variety of popular Mediterranean foods without packing in the carbohydrates, and we promise you won't miss the pita bread! All components of this dish hold up well in the refrigerator so to batch cook, simply double the recipe.

Serves 2

Ingredients:

1 tablespoon oil
¾ pound chicken, cubed
Your favorite seasonings, to taste
1 small cucumber, chopped
10 grape tomatoes, halved
¼ cup thinly sliced red onion
10 kalamata olives, halved
½ cup crumbled feta cheese
½ cup Tzatziki Dipping Sauce (page 265)

Salad Dressing Ingredients:

¼ cup extra-virgin olive oil
1 tablespoon red wine vinegar
1 dollop Dijon mustard
Dried oregano, to taste
Salt and pepper, to taste

Steps:

1. In a pan over medium-high heat, heat oil and cook the chicken on one side until brown, about 4 minutes. Add your favorite seasonings and turn over. Continue to cook until done, around 4 minutes, flipping occasionally.

2. Meanwhile, add the cucumber, tomatoes, onion, olives, and feta cheese to a medium bowl and toss.

3. Whisk all dressing ingredients until thoroughly combined. Pour over the salad and toss until coated.

4. Plate the chicken, salad, and Tzatiki Dipping Sauce, and serve.

Easy Pistachio Avocado Salad

This salad does well on its own, but if you're looking for more protein, chicken is a great addition. The fats from nuts, seeds, avocado, and oil will help you hit your keto macros in the healthiest way possible, and if you prefer to batch prepare this so you have several servings for the week, simply sub kale in for the romaine, as it stands up better after a few days in the fridge, and add the avocado in right before serving.

Serves 2

Salad Ingredients:

1 head romaine lettuce, chopped

3 green onions, chopped, or ¼ cup sliced red onions

½ cup shelled pistachio halves

¼ cup shelled hemp seeds

1 avocado, diced

Dressing Ingredients:

2 tablespoons extra-virgin olive oil

1 tablespoon apple cider vinegar

½ tablespoon coconut aminos

Freshly squeezed lemon, to taste

Steps:

1. Place the chopped romaine in a large bowl.

2. Add the green onions, pistachios, hemp seeds, and avocado.

3. Whisk all dressing ingredients together and thoroughly toss in the salad.

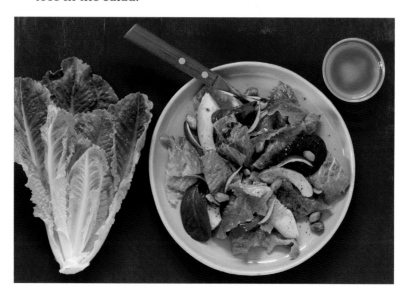

Chicken and Broccoli Alfredo

This dish can be used interchangeably for lunch or dinner, but we included it here because it can be easily packed for lunch and reheated. You won't miss the pasta in this decadent Alfredo dish, and if you want to make it really fast and simple, use already cooked rotisserie chicken.

Serves 4

Ingredients:

1 tablespoon butter

½ cup yellow onions, chopped

2 cloves garlic, minced

1 cup white mushrooms, sliced

1 pound chicken breasts or thighs, cooked and cubed

3 cups broccoli florets, steamed

1½ cups Alfredo sauce (page 262, or store bought)

½ cup shaved Parmesan cheese

1 tablespoon fresh parsley, chopped (optional)

Steps:

1. In a large skillet, melt the butter over medium heat, and add the onions, garlic, and mushrooms. Cook until the onions are translucent and the mushrooms are tender, about 5 minutes. Add the chicken, broccoli, and Alfredo sauce, and combine until evenly coated.

2. Simmer for 3 to 4 minutes, while stirring occasionally.

3. Divide among 4 bowls or sealed containers (if storing for work lunches) and garnish with Parmesan cheese and parsley (optional) before serving.

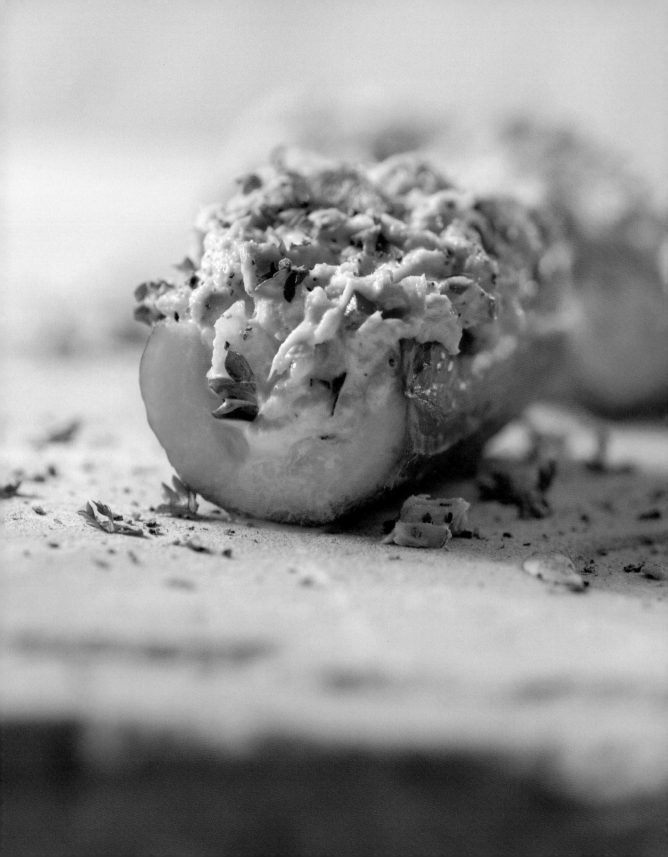

Zucchini Boat Tuna Salad

This is a healthier version of traditional mayo-filled tuna salad, and the handheld zucchini boats make them convenient for a picnic or work lunch. This simple recipe is high in protein and healthy fat and low in carbohydrates, and only takes minutes to prepare.

Serves 1

Ingredients:

1 large zucchini
1 can tuna packed in water, strained
1 tablespoon avocado oil mayo
Juice from ½ lemon
¼ bell pepper, diced
Handful of parsley, chopped
Black pepper, to taste

Steps:

1. Slice the zucchini lengthwise and hollow out by scraping out the inner soft layer and set aside.

2. Mix tuna with avocado oil mayo, lemon juice, and bell pepper.

3. Fill zucchini boat with tuna mixture and top with parsley and ground pepper.

Lunch Snack Pack

Sometimes you don't feel like an actual meal for lunch, and a variety of delicious snacks will do the trick—not to mention, it can be easier and faster to pack and take on the go. For a full week of lunches, simply multiply this recipe by five, package, and refrigerate as it will all hold up for the week.

Ingredients:

1 small container Greek yogurt
4 strawberries
¼ cup raw walnuts
Handful of raw broccoli florets and celery sticks
½ cup mashed avocado for dipping
2 tablespoons peanut butter for dipping
1 hard-boiled egg

Steps:

1. Package all ingredients in a portable container and refrigerate.

Wine Country Lunch Platter

Sometimes it's nice to change it up and have a smorgasbord platter as opposed to a standard hot meal. This is the perfect lunch to introduce your new keto lifestyle to your friends—and you can even enjoy a glass of red wine or two with it!

Serves 1

Ingredients:

4 ounces cooked pork chop, sliced

½ cup chopped or sliced cucumber

1 egg, soft-boiled, halved

1 ounce cheese, sliced

5 olives

1 ounce nuts

¼ cup berries (optional)

Steps:

1. Arrange all ingredients on a platter.

2. Serve with a glass of pinot noir or sauvignon blanc (optional).

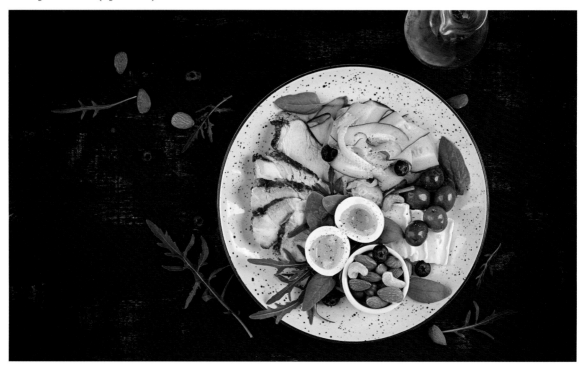

Egg Roll in a Bowl

This dish gives you all of the delicious fillings found in a Chinese egg roll, in one big bowl. Since these bowls keep really well in the refrigerator, this is a great recipe to batch cook ahead of time so you have tasty Chinese food for the week.

Serves 4-6

Ingredients:

2 tablespoons coconut oil
1 medium onion, diced
1 pound ground pork
    sausage
1 pound ground beef
2 teaspoons garlic, minced
⅓ cup low-sodium soy
    sauce
1½ teaspoons ground
    ginger
1½ bags tricolor raw
    coleslaw
3 eggs
Sesame oil for finishing
    (optional)

Steps:

1. In a large pan with coconut oil, sauté the onions for 2 to 3 minutes on medium heat.

2. Add the sausage and beef to the pan and brown, crumbling with a spatula as it cooks for 10 to 12 minutes.

3. Add minced garlic and combine; continue to cook for 1 to 2 minutes.

4. Add soy sauce, ground ginger, and coleslaw.

5. Continue to sauté until you have reached the desired tenderness of the coleslaw.

6. Whisk the eggs in a small bowl, and create a well in the center of the mixture. Pour the eggs in the well and scramble.

7. As the eggs become cooked, combine them with the rest of the mixture.

8. Divide in bowls and drizzle with sesame oil to serve (optional).

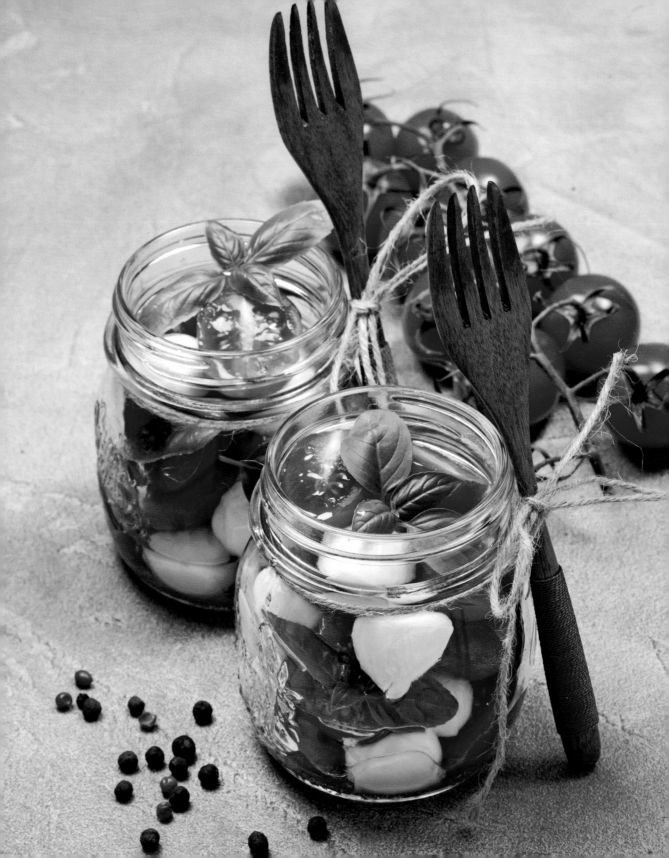

Caprese Salad Jar

If you're in the mood for a fancy Italian dish either at work or on the go, this salad can be made ahead of time as the ingredients hold up well. This vegetarian salad is filling enough for a meal as it's high in protein, but if you're looking for a bit more, grilled chicken is a complementary addition.

Serves 1

Ingredients:

5 mini mozzarella balls
7 cherry tomatoes
Handful fresh basil leaves
1 tablespoon extra-virgin olive oil
½ tablespoon apple cider vinegar
Salt and pepper, to taste

Steps:

1. Slice mozzarella balls and cherry tomatoes in half.

2. Evenly distribute mozzarella, tomatoes, and basil in a jar.

3. Whisk olive oil and apple cider vinegar together and add salt and pepper to taste.

4. Pour over salad and seal with jar lid. Refrigerate until eaten.

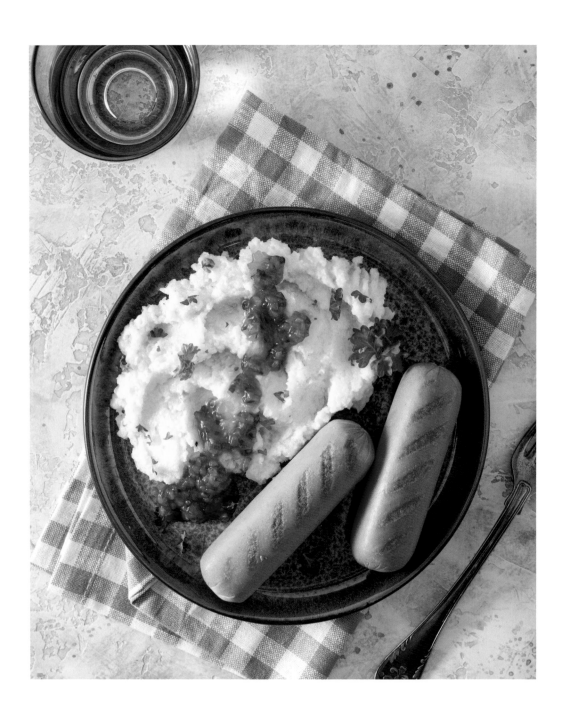

British Bangers and Mash

Yes, we do advise to limit processed meats, but if you're in a pickle for a quick lunch, this is a great option. Not to mention, I thought I would pay homage to my British roots with this one! A tip is to quadruple the mashed cauliflower recipe so you have the tasty low-carb side dish on hand in your refrigerator.

Serves 1

Ingredients:

1 cup cauliflower florets

2 hots dogs or sausages

¼ cup grated Parmesan cheese

Salt and pepper, to taste

Mustard, to garnish (optional)

Sauerkraut, to garnish (optional)

Steps:

1. Steam the cauliflower over medium-high heat until extremely tender, about 20 minutes.

2. Meanwhile, prepare the hot dogs or sausages according to package directions.

3. Once the cauliflower is steamed, mash it in a medium bowl with the grated Parmesan, salt, and pepper until thoroughly combined.

4. Plate the hot dogs or sausages with the mashed cauliflower and garnish with mustard and sauerkraut (optional).

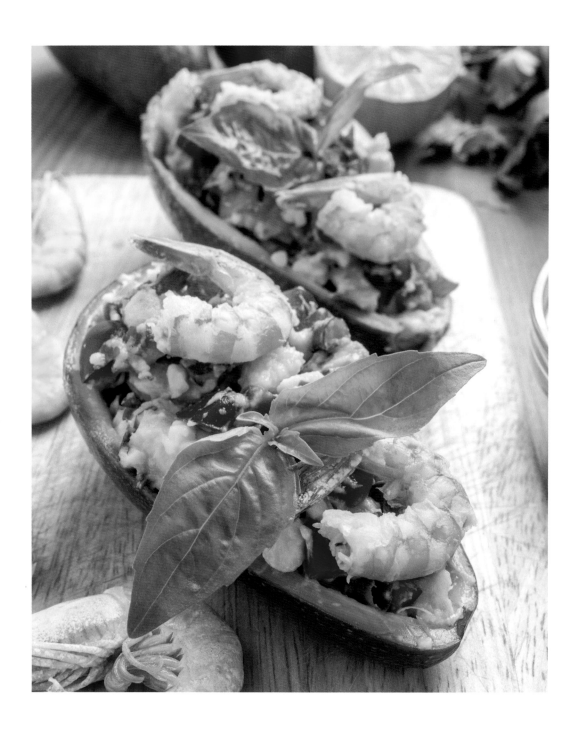

Shrimp and Salsa-Stuffed Avocados

If you're a fan of Mexican food, this recipe has all of the flavors without the carbohydrates, and it's a unique rendition of the typical ceviche dish. The healthy fat and protein found in the avocado and shrimp makes this small meal very filling, or you can use this as an appetizer for a keto-friendly dinner party.

Serves 1

Ingredients:

1 avocado

6 large precooked shrimp, peeled and deveined

1 tablespoon salsa

2 tablespoons shredded Mexican cheese blend

Chopped cilantro, for garnish (optional)

Chopped chives, for garnish (optional)

Steps:

1. Cut the avocado in half, remove pit, and scoop into a small bowl (do not discard the skins). Use a fork to rough chop the avocado into chunks.

2. Rinse the shrimp and chop into bite-size pieces. Place in the bowl with the avocado and add salsa; stir to coat evenly. Add more salsa, to taste, if desired.

3. Add the cheese to the bowl and combine.

4. Scoop the mixture back into the avocado skins for presentation and garnish with cilantro and chives (optional) or scoop into a serving bowl and garnish.

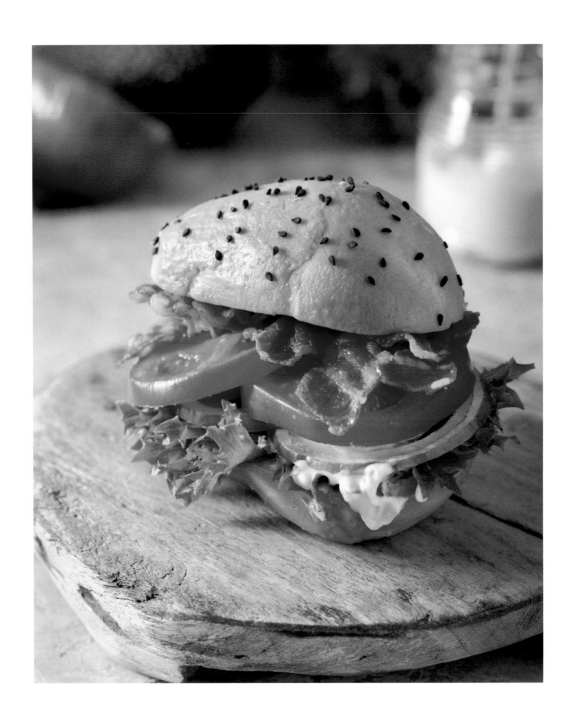

Keto Bacon Lettuce Tomato Avocado Cup

A take on the old BLT sandwich classic, this lettuce cup version employs lots of fresh produce, as well as healthy fats from the avocado and avocado oil mayo. If you want the on-the-go version, simply chop up all ingredients and toss it into a salad!

Serves 1

Ingredients:

2 pieces bacon
3 lettuce leaves
1 tablespoon avocado oil mayo
Sliced red onion, to taste
2 slices tomato
½ avocado

Steps:

1. Cook the bacon over medium heat, turning over occasionally, until cooked through, around 7 minutes.

2. Meanwhile, stack the lettuce leaves on top of each other to create one firm lettuce cup. If you are making a salad, use more than three leaves and chop.

3. Evenly spread the avocado oil mayo on the lettuce cup. If you are making a salad, toss the avocado oil mayo in the chopped lettuce—add more mayo if using extra lettuce.

4. Layer the sliced onion on the lettuce cup, and then layer the tomatoes on top of the onion. If you are making a salad, chop the onion and tomato and toss them into the lettuce.

5. Place the bacon on top of the tomato, and then the avocado on top of the bacon. If you are making a salad, chop the bacon and avocado and toss into the salad.

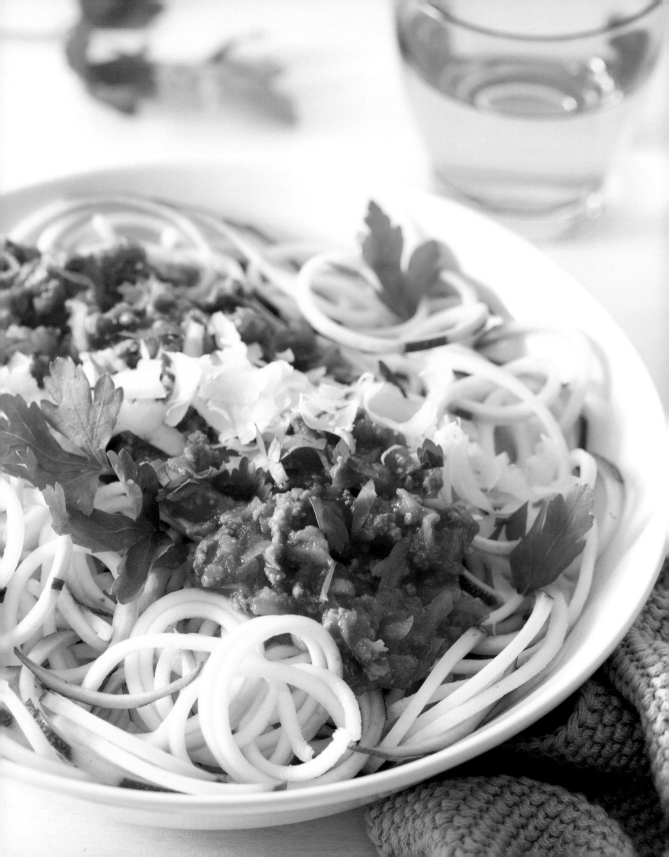

Zoodles Bolognese

If you're in the mood for a traditional pasta dish but want to avoid the excess carbohydrates without sacrificing flavor, this version of spaghetti Bolognese will not disappoint. If you prefer turkey, you can sub that in for the ground beef, or even if you're vegan, you can leave the meat out, and use a nut-based cheese and fresh parsley for the toppers.

Serves 5

Ingredients:

1 tablespoon extra-virgin olive oil

2 pounds ground beef (you can use turkey or chicken if you prefer)

2 cups Low-Carb Pizza & Pasta Sauce (page 263, or store bought)

4 medium zucchini

4 tablespoons freshly chopped parsley

Grated Parmesan cheese, to taste.

Steps:

1. Using extra-virgin olive oil, cook the ground meat in a pan over medium-high heat for 8 minutes until browned on all sides.

2. Add pasta sauce and continue to cook on medium heat for 3 to 5 minutes or until cooked through. Transfer to a bowl when done.

3. While your meat sauce is cooking, use a spiralizer to create your zucchini noodles. If you do not have a spiralizer, you can use a julienne peeler to peel the zucchini all around until you get to the soft center.

4. Using the same meat saucepan, cook the zoodles over medium heat for 3 to 5 minutes until you reach desired tenderness. Add the meat sauce back into the pan and combine with the zoodles or plate the zoodles and top with meat sauce. Top with fresh parsley and grated Parmesan cheese.

Parmesan Kale Salad

This universal salad base will accommodate the favorite toppings of your choice as it pairs nicely with most foods and flavors. The avocado dressing is simple and healthy, and provides a creamy texture that is reminiscent of more decadent salad dressings that sometimes don't have the most ideal ingredients. Diced hard-boiled eggs or chopped steak are complementary additions.

Serves 1

Ingredients:

2 cups curly kale or chopped romaine lettuce

½ avocado

2 tablespoons oil

1 teaspoon apple cider vinegar

1–2 tablespoons grated Parmesan cheese

Freshly squeezed lemon, to taste

Steps:

1. Place the curly kale or romaine in a medium bowl.

2. In a small bowl, mash the avocado with a fork until it has the consistency of paste.

3. Drizzle in the oil gradually as you thoroughly combine with the avocado.

4. Drizzle in the apple cider vinegar and thoroughly combine with the avocado mixture.

5. Using your hands, massage the avocado dressing into the kale or lettuce until all leaves are coated.

6. Top with Parmesan cheese and freshly squeezed lemon, to taste.

Chapter 20

30-Day Keto Dinner Recipes

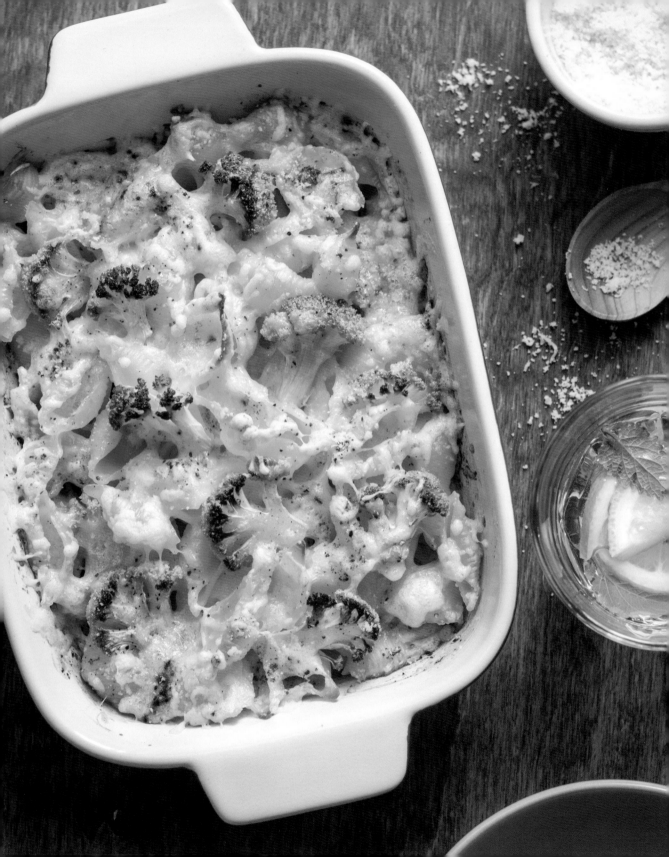

Keto Cauliflower Mac N' Cheese

Mac n' cheese is probably one of the greatest known comfort foods, and you can still work it in while doing keto. While the actual pasta is missing, the flavor and extreme cheesiness is still there and if you're looking for more protein, simply pair this filling side dish with a steak or chicken breast.

Serves 8

Ingredients:

Butter, for baking dish

2 medium heads cauliflower, cut into florets

2 tablespoons avocado oil

Salt, to taste

1 cup heavy cream

6 ounces cream cheese, cubed

4 cups shredded cheddar cheese

2 cups shredded mozzarella

Freshly ground pepper, to taste

¼ cup grated Parmesan

Fresh parsley, chopped (for garnish)

Steps:

1. Preheat oven to 375°F and butter a 9x13-inch baking dish.

2. In a large bowl, toss cauliflower florets with oil and season to taste with salt. Spread cauliflower on two baking sheets and roast until lightly golden, about 40 minutes.

3. While the cauliflower is roasting, heat cream in large pot over medium heat. Bring up to a simmer and then decrease heat to low and stir in all cheeses until melted and combined.

4. Remove from heat and season with ground pepper (and additional salt) as needed.

5. Fold the roasted cauliflower into the cheese mixture and transfer to the prepared baking dish.

6. Bake for about 15 minutes or until golden brown. Top with grated Parmesan and bake for an additional 2 minutes.

7. Garnish with chopped parsley and serve.

Classic Cheeseburger in a Bowl

If you're missing a good old greasy fast food burger, this dish will not disappoint. You'll get all of the classic taste and flavors, even down to the sauce! If you want to turn this bowl into a sandwich, check out the recipes in chapter 8 for your keto-approved cheeseburger bun.

Serves 3

Bowl Ingredients:

1 pound ground beef
½ cup yellow onion, diced
Salt and pepper, to taste
6 cups iceberg or romaine lettuce, shredded
½ cup red onion, sliced
1 cup shredded cheddar cheese
1 cup tomato, diced (optional)
¼ cup dill pickles, sliced or diced

Sauce Ingredients:

¾ cup mayonnaise
2 tablespoons dill pickles, finely minced
1 tablespoon Thousand Island dressing or mustard
½ teaspoon smoked paprika
½ teaspoon garlic powder
½ teaspoon onion powder

Steps:

1. Add the beef to a large pan and brown over medium-high heat for 3 to 4 minutes, breaking up into crumbles.

2. Add the yellow onion, salt, and pepper and continue to cook for 4 to 5 minutes or until the onion is softened and the beef is browned and cooked through.

3. Meanwhile, whisk all sauce ingredients in a medium bowl until combined.

4. Divide lettuce into 3 bowls, then top each bowl with ⅓ of the browned beef, onion, cheese, tomato (optional), and pickles.

5. To serve, drizzle with sauce.

Addicting Slow Cooker Cheesy Chicken

The name of this dish may sound a little strange, but this is quite the popular dish in the keto community. If you're tired of standard chicken recipes, you may want to try this as it's gooey and cheesy, with bacon added. This dish is filling on its own or can be paired with a crisp green salad.

Serves 6

Ingredients:

½ cup bone broth or chicken stock

1 tablespoon dried parsley

2 teaspoons dried dill

1 teaspoon dried chives

½ teaspoon onion powder

¼ teaspoon garlic powder

2 pounds boneless, skinless chicken breasts

Salt and pepper, to taste

2 (8 ounce) blocks cream cheese, cubed

2¼ cup shredded cheddar cheese, divided

8 slices cooked bacon, crumbled

Chopped chives, for serving

Steps:

1. Pour the chicken broth into a slow cooker and combine with dried parsley, dill, chives, onion powder, and garlic powder.

2. Add half the chicken and season with salt and pepper, to taste. Repeat with the remainder of the chicken.

3. Stir the broth to coat the chicken and set the slow cooker on low for 6 hours or on high for 2 hours.

4. Using two forks, shred the chicken while it remains in the slow cooker. Stir in the cream cheese and 2 cups of the shredded cheddar cheese until melted.

5. To serve, top with remaining cheddar cheese, bacon, and chives.

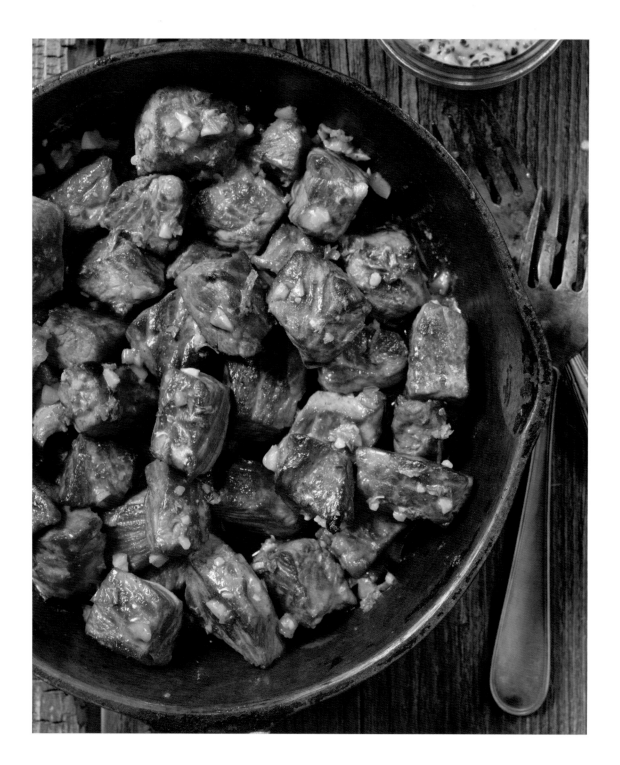

Garlic Butter Steak Bites

This is a unique and simple way to prepare your steak, and so many variations can be created from this easy base recipe by adding your own seasonings and flavors. Steak bites are delicious with a trio of dips—mashed avocado, avocado oil mayo, and Tzatziki Dipping Sauce (page 265) are our favorites, or you can pair with a side salad with ranch dressing.

Serves 4

Ingredients:

2 pounds ribeye steak
Salt and pepper, to taste
4 tablespoons oil, divided
4 tablespoons butter, divided
2 large garlic cloves, minced, divided
1 teaspoon fresh parsley leaves, minced

Steps:

1. Cut steak into ¾-inch cubes and season with salt and pepper.

2. Heat half of the oil in a large skillet over medium-high heat. Add half the steak in a single layer and cook, turning a few times until golden and medium rare, about 5 minutes.

3. Add half of the butter and half of the garlic and toss to coat.

4. Remove steak to a serving bowl. Repeat with remaining steak.

5. Garnish steak with parsley.

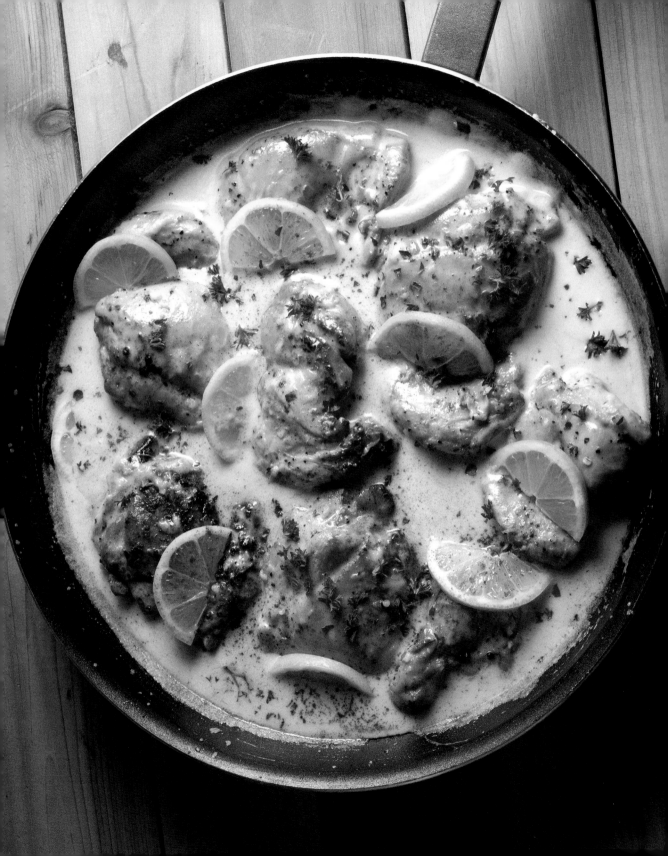

Creamy Keto Chicken Piccata

Chicken piccata is typically dredged in flour, but you can still get all the flavor without the added step (or the carbohydrates) of the dredging. This rendition of the old Italian classic has a keto spin with added cream for a more decadent sauce.

Serves 2-3

Ingredients:

Your favorite seasonings
6 chicken thighs
2 garlic cloves, minced
2 tablespoons oil, divided
2 tablespoons butter, divided
¼ cup onions, finely chopped
½ cup chicken broth
Juice of 2 lemons
3 tablespoons capers
½ cup cream
Salt and pepper, to taste
Chopped parsley for serving

Steps:

1. Season the chicken thighs to taste, and then rub them with the minced garlic.

2. Heat half the oil and half of the butter in a large pan and add the chicken thighs. Cook on each side for 6 minutes or until you have reached an internal temperature of 165°F. Remove to a plate and set aside.

3. In the same pan, add the remaining oil and butter over medium heat. Add the onions and sauté for 2 to 3 minutes. Add the chicken broth and increase to high heat, letting the broth simmer until it has reduced to about half, around 4 minutes.

4. Lower the heat to medium and add the lemon juice and mix. Then add the capers, cream, and salt and pepper, to taste.

5. Place the cooked chicken back in the pan and spoon the sauce over the chicken, cooking for 2 more minutes. Add parsley to garnish.

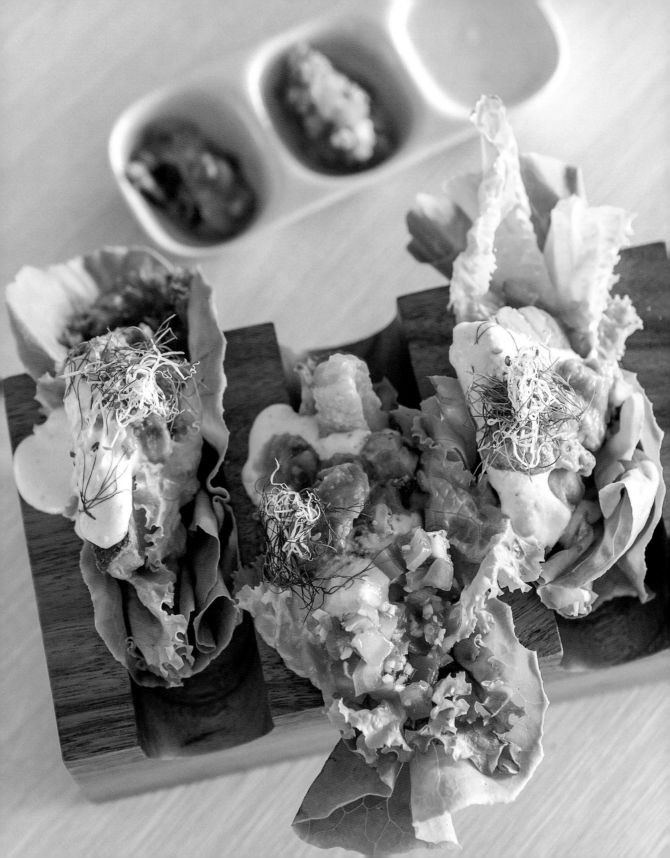

Simple Salmon Taco Lettuce Wraps

This simple recipe is light and refreshing but filled with flavor. Reminiscent of traditional seaside cuisine, the healthy fats will keep you satisfied while the low-glycemic carbohydrates will provide antioxidants and fiber. Brighten these wraps up by squeezing fresh lime on top.

Serves 2

Ingredients:

1 tablespoon avocado oil
1 pound wild salmon
Salt and pepper, to taste
1 head butter lettuce
1 avocado, mashed
2 tablespoons Greek yogurt
2 tablespoons pico de gallo
    or salsa
1 lemon, halved

Steps:

1. Heat the oil in a medium pan and add the salmon.

2. Add salt and pepper to taste, and cook over medium heat until cooked through, around 12 minutes. Break the salmon apart while cooking—leaving the skin on or removing is optional.

3. Display the lettuce, mashed avocado, Greek yogurt, salsa, and lemon. Assemble the tacos by scooping the cooked salmon into individual lettuce cups and topping with taco add-ons, and freshly squeezed lemon.

Roasted Salmon Stuffed with Spinach Artichoke Dip

If you're a fan of lox and cream cheese, you'll love this roasted rendition. Even if salmon isn't your favorite, give this a try—the cream cheese tones it down, making it taste like a more mild whitefish.

Serves 4

Ingredients:

4 (6–8 ounce) salmon fillets
1 batch Spinach Artichoke
    Dip (page 251)
Olive oil for drizzling
Salt and pepper, to taste
Fresh lemon for serving

Steps:

1. Preheat the oven to 400°F.

2. Make a 2- to 3-inch incision in the middle of each fillet and stuff with 2 to 3 tablespoons Spinach Artichoke Dip. Drizzle the top of the salmon with olive oil and salt and pepper to taste.

3. Roast until cooked through, around 20 minutes.

4. Top with freshly squeezed lemon and store extra dip in the refrigerator for up to 10 days.

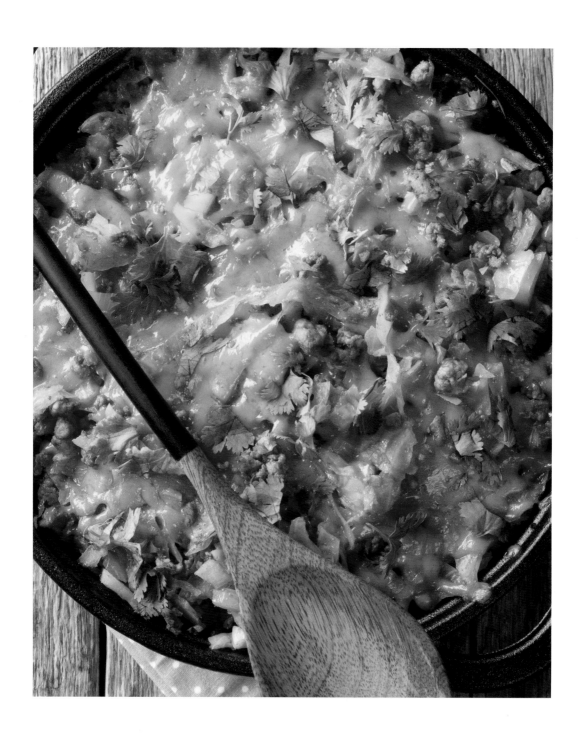

Cheesy Beef Cabbage Roll Casserole

This is a casserole take on the classic cabbage roll dish, but it has some added cheese for a rich and creamy texture. To batch cook, simply double, triple, or even quadruple this recipe as this casserole is freezer friendly. Serve warm with a small arugula salad.

Serves 4–5

Ingredients:

2 pounds ground beef
4 cups cabbage, shredded
½ yellow onion, thinly sliced
¾ cup sour cream
2 teaspoons garlic powder
Salt and pepper, to taste
1 cup shredded cheddar cheese, divided
Cilantro for garnish (optional)

Steps:

1. Preheat oven to 400°F.

2. In large pan over medium-high heat, brown the ground beef, while breaking into pieces with a spatula for 3 to 4 minutes.

3. Add the cabbage and onion and combine; continue to cook for 5 to 6 minutes while stirring and breaking up the beef.

4. Remove from heat and add in sour cream, stirring until combined. Add the garlic powder, salt, pepper, and half of the shredded cheddar cheese while mixing.

5. Pour into a baking dish and bake for 30 minutes. Top with the remainder of the shredded cheese and return to the oven until cheese is melted and browned, around 5 minutes. Garnish with cilantro (optional).

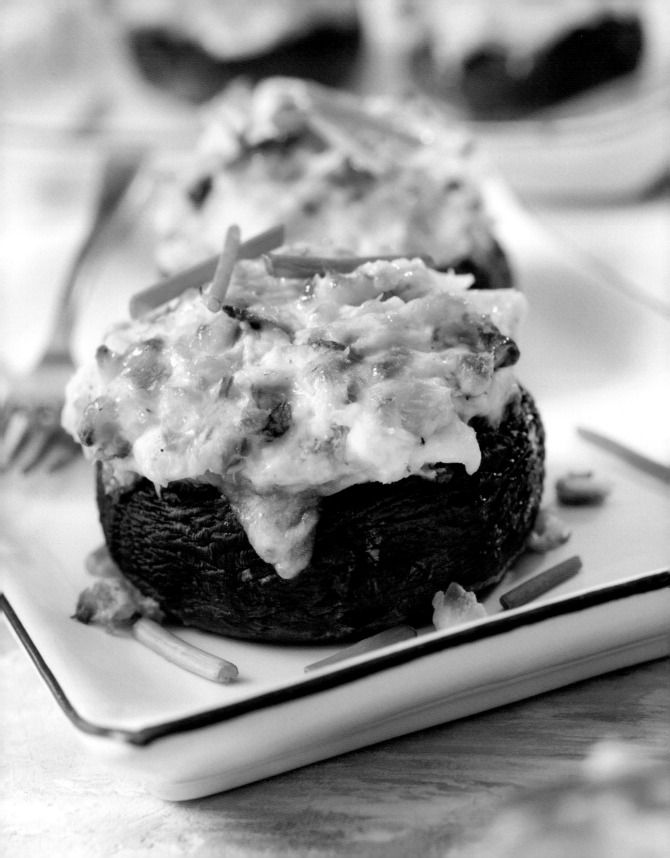

Creamy Crab Stuffed Mushrooms

These stuffed mushrooms may strike you as a fancy party appetizer but they are simple to make and when paired with a side salad or green vegetables, your meal is complete. Feel free to use canned crab if you can't find it fresh, or if you prefer shrimp, the small bay variety works wonderfully in the dish.

Serves 4

Ingredients:

20 ounces cremini mushrooms (20-25 individual mushrooms)

4 ounces cream cheese, room temperature

4 ounces crabmeat, finely chopped

5 cloves garlic, minced

1 teaspoon dried oregano

½ teaspoon paprika

½ teaspoon black pepper

¼ teaspoon salt

2 tablespoons finely grated Parmesan cheese

1 tablespoon chopped chives or parsley

Steps:

1. Preheat the oven to 400°F. Prepare a baking sheet lined with parchment paper.

2. Snap stems from mushrooms, discarding the stems and placing the mushroom caps on the baking sheet 1 inch apart from each other.

3. In a large mixing bowl, combine the cream cheese, crabmeat, garlic, oregano, paprika, pepper, and salt. Stir until well-mixed without any lumps of cream cheese.

4. Stuff the mushroom caps with the mixture. Evenly sprinkle Parmesan cheese on top of the stuffed mushrooms.

5. Bake until the mushrooms are very tender and the stuffing is nicely browned on top, about 30 minutes. Top with chives and serve while hot.

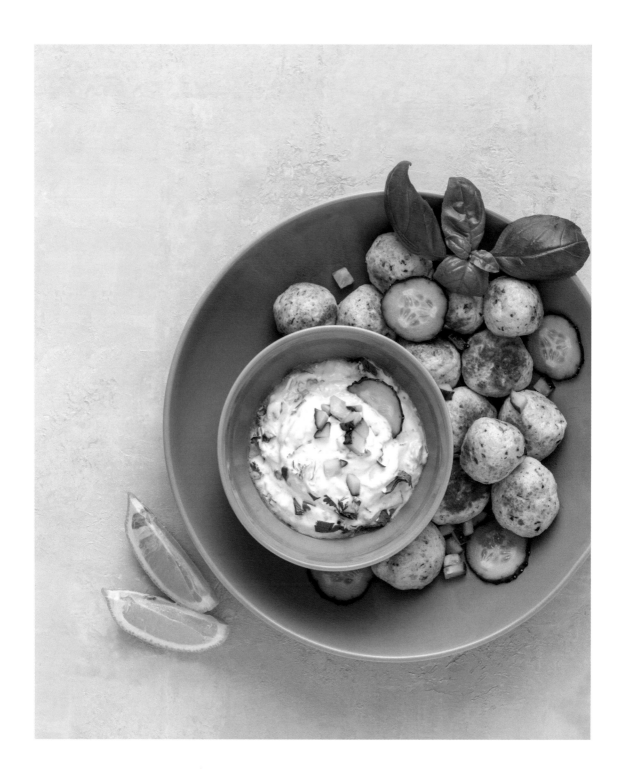

Mediterranean Meatballs

These Greek meatballs have a different flavor profile than that of their Italian counterparts so if you're looking for something a little different, this is for you. Even without the typical breadcrumb filler, these meatballs are tender and fluffy, and even that much more decadent when paired with Tzatziki Dipping Sauce.

Serves 4

Ingredients:

2 pounds ground chicken
8 ounces feta cheese, grated or crumbled
1 lemon, zested
1 tablespoon lemon juice
2 tablespoons rosemary, finely chopped
1 egg
1 teaspoon black pepper
½ teaspoon salt
1 tablespoon olive oil
1 tablespoon butter

Steps:

1. In a bowl place all the ingredients, except the oil and butter, and combine thoroughly with hands.

2. Roll the mixture into about 30 evenly sized meatballs.

3. Heat a large nonstick frying pan over medium heat and add the oil and butter.

4. Place the meatballs into the frying pan and cook for 7 minutes on each side; reduce heat if meatballs start to brown too quickly.

5. Remove from the pan and serve with Tzatziki Dipping Sauce (page 265).

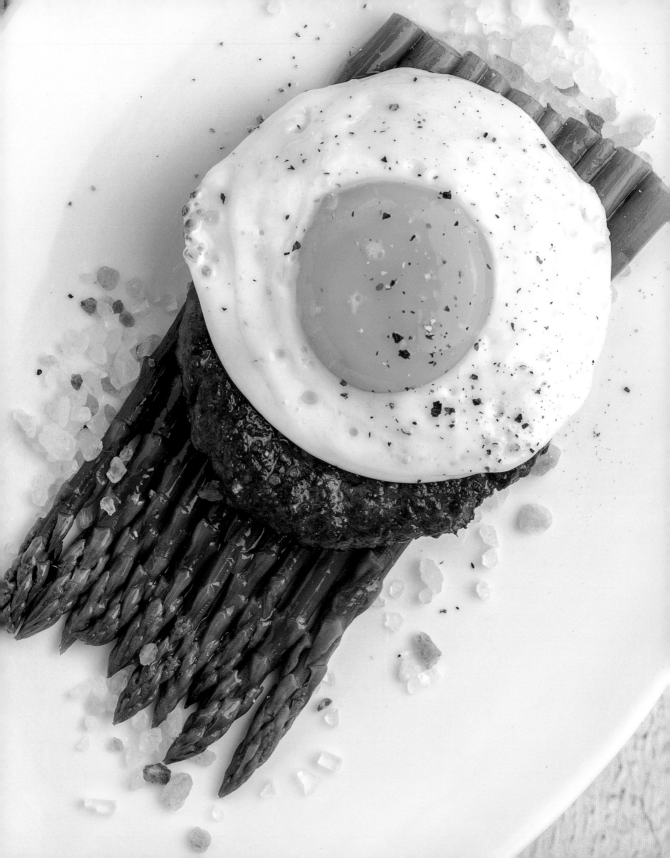

Egg-Sparagus Burger

This combination brings two different concepts together—the trendy restaurant's sautéed asparagus topped with fried egg along with a good old fashioned burger. The egg yolk provides a delicious sauce for this combination, however, feel free to add mayonnaise, cheese, avocado, tomato, and onion.

Serves 1

Ingredients:

½ pound ground beef, divided
Your favorite seasonings
6–8 asparagus spears
1 tablespoon oil
1 egg
Salt and pepper, to taste

Steps:

1. Form the ground beef into a patty and season to taste.

2. Cook in a small pan over medium-high heat until browned on one side, about 5 minutes.

3. Flip over and continue to cook until you have reached an internal temperature of 150°F, around 8 more minutes.

4. Meanwhile, sauté the asparagus in oil over medium heat, flipping occasionally until cooked through, around 8 to 12 minutes depending on thickness.

5. Panfry a sunny-side-up egg in a separate pan.

6. Plate the asparagus, followed by the burger, and top the burger with the egg. Add salt and pepper to taste.

Mediterranean Chicken Pesto Casserole

Between the Mediterranean superstars, the olives, feta cheese, and pesto pack this creamy chicken dish with flavor, and it's simple to make. A crisp side salad makes the perfect pairing to this comfort food dish.

Serves 4

Ingredients:

1½ pounds chicken breasts or boneless chicken thighs

Salt and pepper, to taste

2 tablespoons butter or ghee

5 tablespoons pesto (page 273, or store bought)

1¼ cups heavy cream

3 ounces pitted olives

5 ounces feta cheese, crumbled

1 garlic clove, minced

Fresh parsley for garnish

Steps:

1. Preheat oven to 400°F.

2. Cut the chicken into bite-size pieces and season with salt and pepper.

3. Add butter or ghee to a large skillet with the chicken and cook over medium-high heat, until browned on all sides, but not all of the way cooked through.

4. Combine the pesto and heavy cream in a bowl.

5. Add the chicken, olives, feta cheese, and garlic to a baking dish. Add the pesto/cream mixture.

6. Bake in the oven until the dish turns bubbly and light brown around the edges, around 25 minutes. Garnish with fresh parsley before serving.

Shirataki Carbonara

This carbonara rendition is a keto-revised take on the old classic. Even if your family isn't following the same keto plan, they will be sure to love this rich and creamy pasta dish. If you can't find shirataki noodles at your local grocery store, zoodles (zucchini noodles) work well as a substitution.

Serves 2

Ingredients:

4 slices bacon

3 ounces chicken breast

1 (7-ounce) packet shirataki noodles

1 large egg yolk

2–3 tablespoons Parmesan cheese

1 cup heavy whipping cream

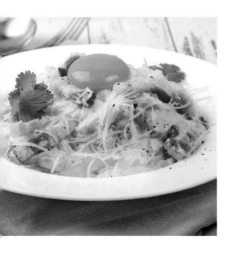

Steps:

1. Dice the bacon and cook over medium heat until it cooks through but does not get crispy. Remove from pan and set aside.

2. Dice the chicken and cook over medium heat in the same pan as the bacon, until almost fully cooked, around 6 minutes. Remove the chicken and set aside.

3. Meanwhile, cook (using a dry frying pan with no oil or butter) the shirataki noodles so that all excess water evaporates, around 7 minutes.

4. In a small bowl, thoroughly combine the egg yolk and Parmesan cheese until you have a smooth paste.

5. In the same pan used for the bacon and chicken, add half of the cream and add the Parmesan egg mixture and combine over medium heat. This may take a few minutes until it is smooth.

6. Add the remaining cream, chicken, and bacon and incorporate.

7. Combine the chicken-bacon sauce with the noodles and serve hot.

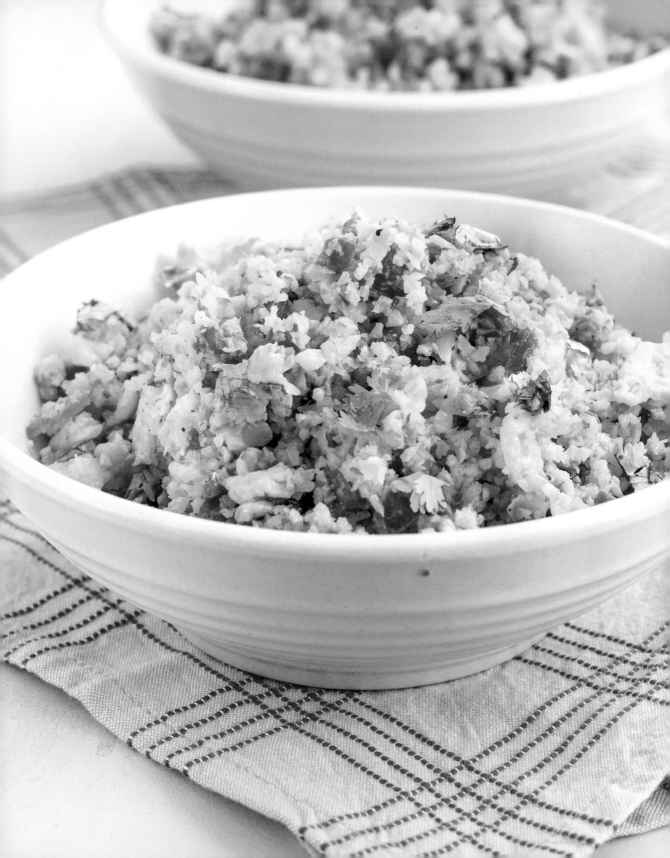

Cauliflower Fried Rice

If you're in the mood for Chinese food, this recipe will still keep your macros in line to get results. You can add any protein you choose to make it a complete meal or feel free to have it on its own. Chicken, shrimp, or chunks of salmon are complementary additions to this dish.

Serves 3

Ingredients:

3 eggs
1 tablespoon coconut oil
1 tablespoon sesame oil
½ small onion, diced
5 scallions, diced
½ cup diced red bell pepper
2 garlic cloves, minced
20 ounces riced cauliflower (store bought is okay)
3 tablespoons soy sauce, or more to taste
1 teaspoon ginger powder
1 tablespoon coconut aminos

Steps:

1. Crack eggs into a small bowl and beat with a fork.

2. Heat a large sauté pan or wok over medium heat with coconut oil. Add the eggs and cook, turning a few times until set; set aside on a plate.

3. In the same pan, add the sesame oil and sauté onion, scallions, bell pepper, and garlic about 4 to 5 minutes, or until soft. Raise the heat to medium-high.

4. Add the riced cauliflower to the sauté pan along with soy sauce, ginger, and coconut aminos. Mix, cover, and cook 5 to 6 minutes, stirring frequently, until the cauliflower is slightly crispy on the outside but tender on the inside.

5. Add the scrambled eggs and combine and remove from heat to serve.

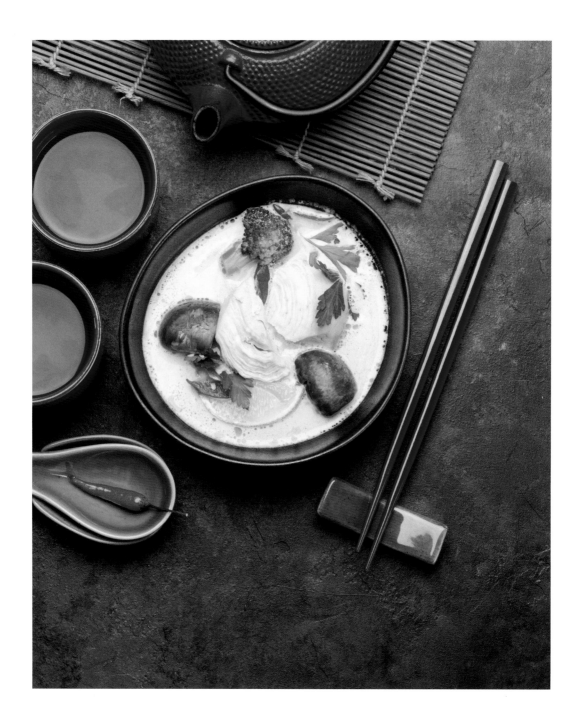

Tom Kha Thai Soup

Although this is just a soup, it's aromatic, silky, and a complete meal in one blow with lots of filling ingredients. If you're looking for a completely different chicken and broccoli dish, this one is sure to do the trick.

Serves 4–6

Ingredients:

2 cups broccoli florets, chopped into bite-size pieces

2 stalks fresh lemongrass, tough outer layers removed

1-inch piece ginger, peeled

1 tablespoon lime zest

¼ cup lime juice

6 cups low-sodium chicken broth

1½ pounds skinless, boneless chicken thighs, cut into 1-inch pieces

8 ounces shiitake or oyster mushrooms, stemmed and cut into bite-size pieces

1 (13.5-ounce) can coconut milk

2 tablespoons fish sauce

1 tablespoon coconut aminos

Cilantro leaves and lime wedges for serving

Red jalapeño pepper, very thinly sliced for serving (optional)

Steps:

1. Over high heat, steam the broccoli until slightly tender, around 12 minutes.

2. Meanwhile, using the back of a knife, lightly smash lemongrass and ginger; cut lemongrass into 4-inch pieces.

3. Bring lemongrass, ginger, lime zest, lime juice, and broth to a boil in a large saucepan. Reduce heat and simmer until flavors are melded, around 8 to 10 minutes.

4. Strain broth into clean saucepan; discard solids.

5. Add chicken and return to a boil. Reduce heat, add mushrooms, and simmer, stirring occasionally, until chicken is cooked through and mushrooms are soft, around 20 to 25 minutes.

6. Mix in coconut milk, fish sauce, and coconut aminos.

7. Serve with cilantro leaves, lime wedges, and jalapeño pepper (optional).

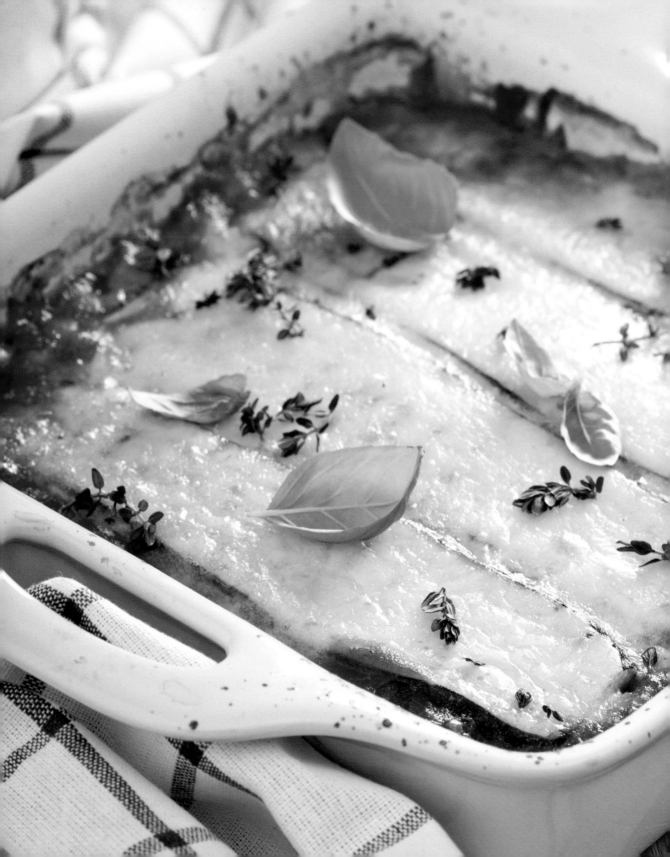

Zucchini Lasagna Bolognese

This low-carbohydrate lasagna is still prepared similarly to the hearty favorite, using the same method but with zucchini strips instead of pasta. This filling dish will satisfy on its own or can be paired with a side salad, topped with Italian dressing.

Serves 5

Ingredients:

1 pound zucchini (about 3 medium)

3 tablespoons extra-virgin olive oil, divided

Salt, to taste

4 cloves garlic, minced

2 pounds ground beef

2 cups tomato or spaghetti sauce

12 ounces full-fat ricotta cheese

½ cup grated Parmesan cheese

1 large egg

3 cups mozzarella cheese, shredded

Steps:

1. Preheat the oven to 400°F. Line a large baking sheet with parchment paper.

2. Use a mandoline or knife to slice zucchini lengthwise into thin sheets, about ¼-inch thick. Arrange zucchini on the baking sheet, in a single layer. Brush both sides with olive oil (use about 2 tablespoons), then sprinkle both sides lightly with sea salt. Roast for 15 to 20 minutes, until soft and mostly dry.

3. When done, remove the zucchini from the oven but leave it on at 400. Pat the zucchini with paper towels to soak up any extra water or oil.

4. Heat the remaining tablespoon of oil in a sauté pan on the stove over medium-high heat. Add the garlic and sauté for 30 to 60 seconds, until fragrant. Add the ground beef. Cook for about 10 minutes, until browned. Stir in the sauce and remove from heat. Taste and adjust salt/pepper if needed.

5. Combine the ricotta and Parmesan cheeses. Stir in the egg.

6. Arrange a layer of zucchini slices at the bottom of a 9x13-inch glass casserole dish. Top with half of the meat sauce. Dollop small pieces of the ricotta cheese mixture (using half of the total amount), then spread. Finally top with half of the shredded mozzarella. Repeat the layers a second time, with shredded mozzarella last on top.

7. Bake for 15 minutes, until the cheese on top is melted and golden. Garnish with fresh basil, if desired.

Easy-Bake Lemon Butter Fish

If you are newer to seafood, this is a wonderful recipe to try as it has a very mild fish taste—if you like chicken, you will probably enjoy this dish! Mild whitefish pairs well with steamed or sautéed green beans, with a generous amount of freshly squeezed lemon on top. To brighten it up even more, add some more fresh herbs in addition to the parsley.

Serves 4

Ingredients:

¼ cup melted butter
4 garlic cloves, minced
Zest and juice of 1 lemon
2 tablespoons fresh parsley, minced
Salt and pepper, to taste
4 fillets of cod, halibut, or rockfish
1 lemon, sliced

Steps:

1. Preheat oven to 425°F.

2. In a bowl, combine the butter, garlic, lemon zest, lemon juice, and parsley; season with salt and pepper to taste.

3. Place the fish in a greased baking dish. Pour the lemon butter mixture over the fish and top with fresh lemon slices. Bake for 12 to 15 minutes, or until fish is flaky and cooked through.

4. Serve the fish topped with fresh parsley and freshly squeezed lemon juice.

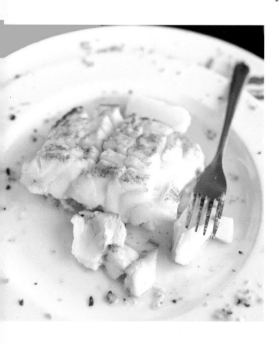

Chapter 21

30-Day Keto Side Dishes, Snacks, Dressings & Sauces

Cauliflower Hummus

Serves 4

Ingredients:

1 medium head cauliflower

4 tablespoons extra-virgin olive oil

½ cup tahini

2 garlic cloves

⅓ cup lemon juice

1 teaspoon salt

½ teaspoon ground black pepper

Chopped fresh parsley, to taste (optional)

Steps:

1. Preheat oven to 375°F and chop cauliflower into small florets.

2. Toss in extra-virgin olive oil and place on a baking sheet; roast until tender, about 20 minutes.

3. Place the roasted cauliflower in a food processor or blender and combine with all other ingredients.

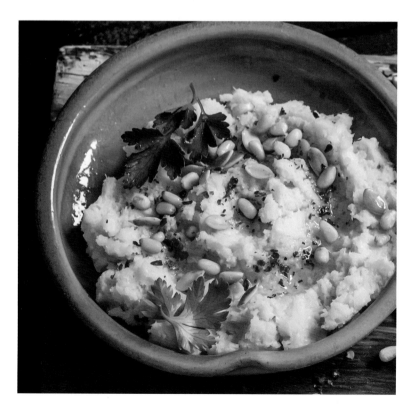

Asparagus in Gorgonzola Sauce

Serves 2

Ingredients:

10 asparagus spears
Gorgonzola sauce
(page 265)

Steps:

1. Steam the asparagus spears until tender, around 10 minutes.

2. Top with Gorgonzola sauce.

Spinach Artichoke Dip

Makes 2 cups

Ingredients:

1 (9-ounce) box frozen spinach, defrosted
14 ounces canned artichoke hearts
8 ounces cream cheese
¼ cup sour cream
1 teaspoon garlic powder
Salt and pepper, to taste
½ teaspoon red pepper flakes (optional)
1 cup mozzarella

Steps:

1. Place defrosted spinach and artichokes in a colander and press firmly to extract as much liquid as possible, and set aside.

2. Add cream cheese to a medium microwave-safe bowl and soften in the microwave for 30 seconds or until the cream cheese is the same consistency as mayonnaise.

3. Add spinach, artichokes, sour cream, garlic powder, salt and pepper, and red pepper flakes (optional) and combine.

4. Fold in the mozzarella cheese.

5. Refrigerate for at least one hour and serve with vegetables to dip or as a steak topper or baked salmon or chicken stuffer.

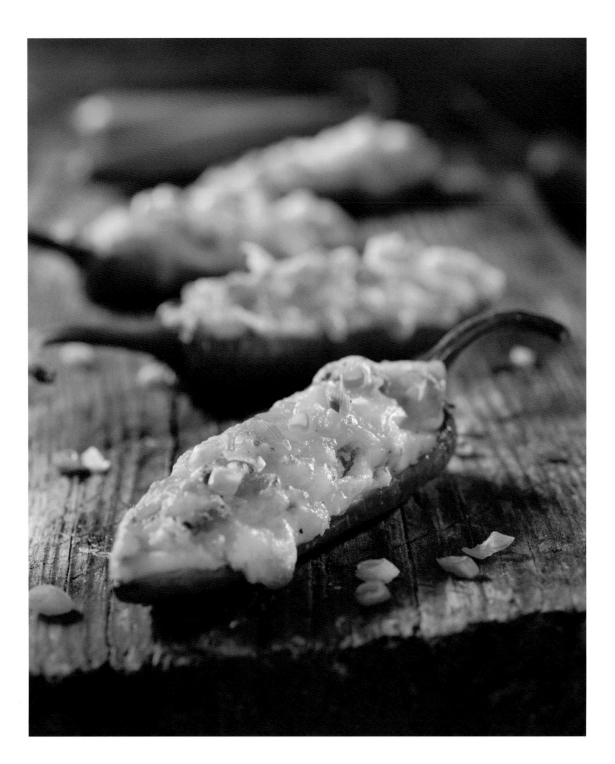

Jalapeño Poppers

Serves 3

Ingredients:

5 slices bacon
6 jalapeño peppers
3 ounces cream cheese, softened
¼ cup shredded cheddar cheese
½ teaspoon garlic powder

Steps:

1. Preheat oven to 400°F.

2. In pan over medium heat, cook the bacon until crispy, around 10 minutes, flipping over occasionally. Chop and set aside.

3. Meanwhile, line a baking sheet with parchment paper.

4. Slice the jalapeños in half, lengthwise, and remove inner seeds and membranes.

5. In a medium bowl combine the cream cheese, cheddar cheese, garlic powder, and cooked bacon.

6. Spoon the cheese mixture into each jalapeño half and place the filled peppers, cheese-side up, on the lined baking sheet.

7. Bake for 18 to 20 minutes until the cheese is melted and slightly crisp on top.

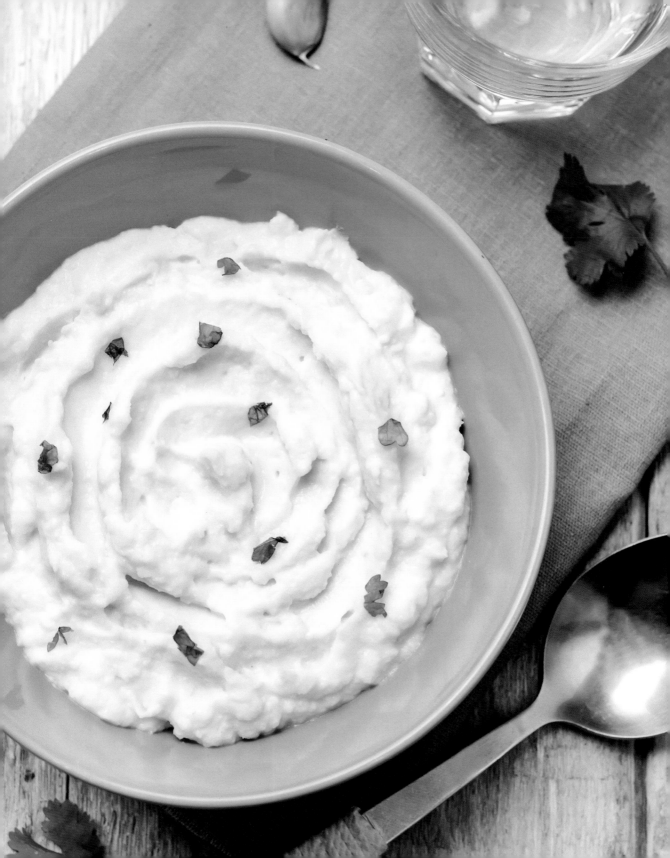

Mashed Cauliflower

Serves 4

Ingredients:

1 head cauliflower
½ cup grated Parmesan cheese
Salt and pepper, to taste

Steps:

1. Chop cauliflower and steam until extremely tender.

2. Using a potato masher or fork, mash into a mashed-potato texture.

3. Add grated Parmesan and thoroughly combine. Season with salt and pepper, to taste.

Creamy Spinach Soup

Makes 5 cups

Ingredients:

3 cups raw spinach
3 garlic cloves, minced
2 tablespoons butter or ghee
1½ cups bone broth or vegetable broth
1 cup heavy cream
1 cup shredded mozzarella cheese (optional)

Steps:

1. Over medium heat in a large pan, sauté the spinach and garlic in butter until the spinach is wilted, around 5 minutes.

2. Add the bone broth and cream and combine.

3. Transfer to a blender and blend for 2 to 3 minutes.

4. Transfer back to the pan until the soup boils.

5. Add the mozzarella cheese and stir until melted (optional).

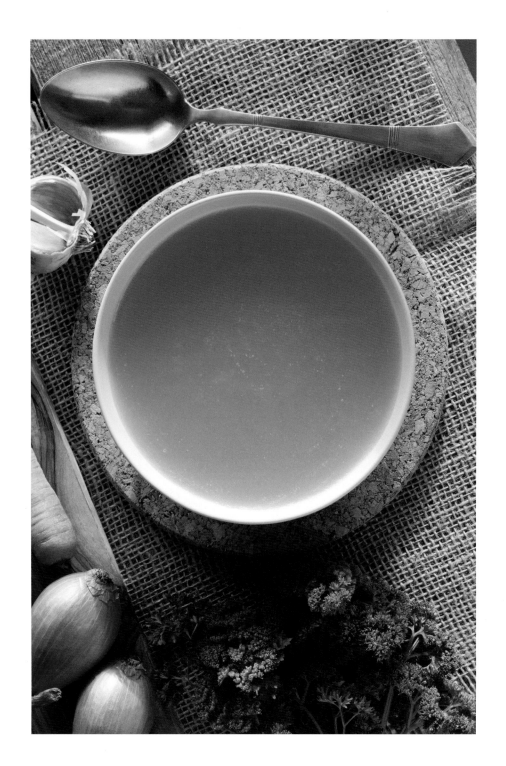

Bone Broth

Serves 4

Ingredients:

1 gallon water
2 tablespoons apple cider vinegar
2-4 pounds animal bones
Salt and pepper, to taste

Steps:

1. Place all ingredients in a large pot or slow cooker.

2. Bring to a boil.

3. Reduce to a simmer and cook for 12-24 hours. The longer it cooks, the better it will taste and more nutritious it will be.

4. Allow the broth to cool. Strain it into a large container and discard the solids.

Four-Ingredient Salmon Dip

Makes 2 cups

Ingredients:

8 ounces smoked salmon, finely chopped
8 ounces crème fraîche
Juice from 2 lemons
1-2 tablespoons fresh dill, finely chopped

Steps:

1. In a medium bowl, combine the salmon and crème fraîche until the crème fraîche turns pink.

2. Add the lemon juice and dill and mix until thoroughly incorporated.

3. Serve with endive leaves or radish slices to dip.

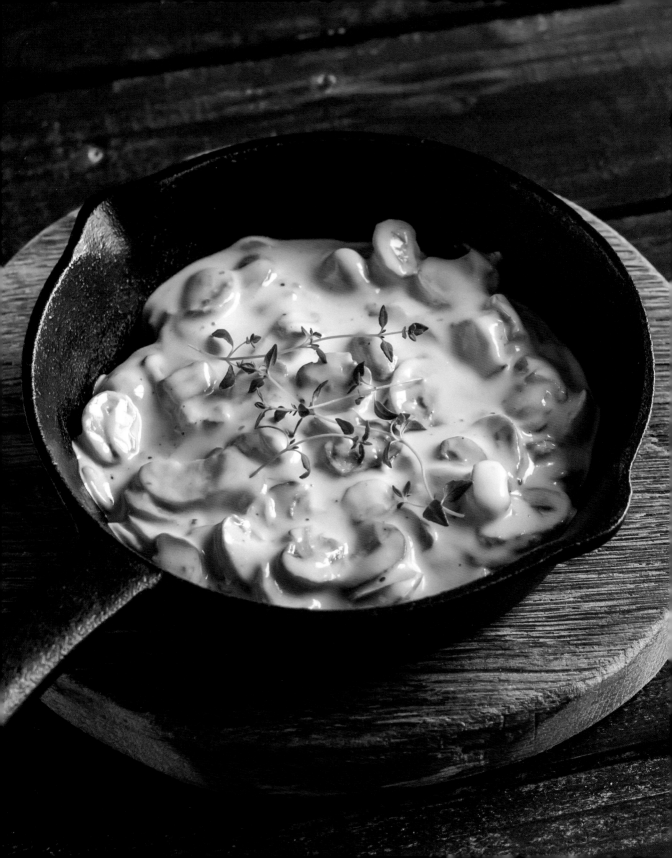

Mushroom Stroganoff

Serves 6

Mushroom Ingredients:

4 cups mushrooms, sliced
3 cloves garlic, minced
½ yellow onion, thinly sliced
3 tablespoons extra-virgin olive oil
3 tablespoons tamari
¼ cup white wine

Stroganoff Sauce Ingredients:

2 tablespoons extra-virgin olive oil
1 tablespoon sun-dried tomatoes
1 tablespoon paprika
½ cup vegetable stock
½ cup cashews
1 teaspoon rosemary
1 teaspoon thyme
1 teaspoon black pepper

Steps:

1. Toss sliced mushrooms, garlic, and onion together in the olive oil and tamari. Set aside and marinate for 10 to 15 minutes.

2. Pan-cook mushroom mixture in a skillet over medium heat until tender; add wine and simmer for 5 minutes.

3. In a food processor or blender, combine extra-virgin olive oil, sun-dried tomatoes, paprika, vegetable stock, cashews, rosemary, thyme, and pepper until smooth.

4. Transfer into the pan with mushrooms and continue to simmer until sauce thickens.

5. Serve on its own as a side dish or as a protein topping.

Parmesan Roasted Fennel

Serves 2

Ingredients:

1 large fennel bulb, quartered and stems removed
1 tablespoon extra-virgin olive oil
2 tablespoons grated Parmesan cheese

Steps:

1. Boil or steam the quartered fennel until tender; toss in extra-virgin olive oil.

2. Roast for 10 minutes at 400°F; sprinkle with Parmesan cheese and roast for 2 additional minutes.

Creamy Cucumber Salad

Serves 2

Ingredients:

½ cup plain almond or
    coconut yogurt

1 green onion, chopped

1 tablespoon sliced red onion

Black pepper to taste

1 tablespoon fresh dill,
    chopped (or ½ teaspoon
    dried)

1 garlic clove, minced

½ cup cucumber, thinly
    sliced

Steps:

1. Combine yogurt with green onion, red onion, pepper, dill, and garlic.

2. Add cucumber slices and toss until evenly coated.

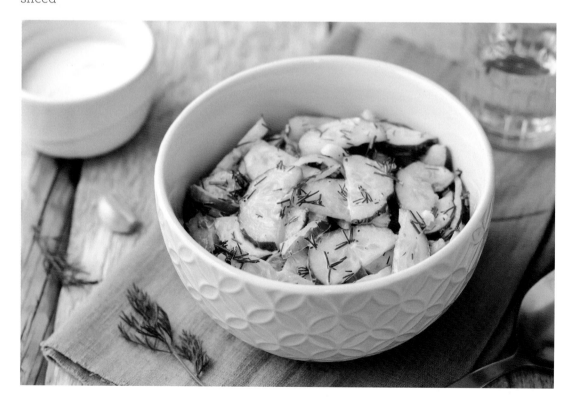

Zucchini Chips

Serves 4

Ingredients:

2 medium zucchini
1 tablespoon oil
Salt, to taste
Your favorite seasonings,
   to taste (optional)

Steps:

1. Preheat oven to 200°F. Line 2 baking sheets with parchment paper.

2. Cut the zucchini into ⅛-inch slices (a mandoline works well).

3. Toss the zucchini slices in oil, salt, and your favorite seasonings.

4. Place the slices side by side (they can touch but not overlap) and bake for about 2½ hours, rotating the pans halfway through.

5. The chips are done when they are golden and just starting to get crispy. Allow them to cool in the oven with the heat off and the door propped slightly open.

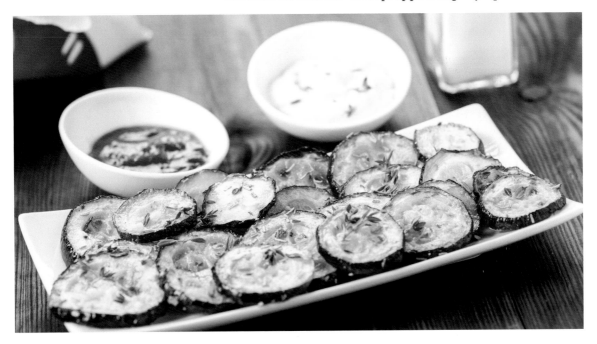

Dressings and Sauces

Creamy Alfredo Sauce

Serves 4

Ingredients:

⅓ cup butter
2 cloves garlic, minced
4 ounces cream cheese,
  cubed
1 cup half-and-half
½ cup grated Parmesan
  cheese
½ teaspoon dried oregano
½ teaspoon salt
½ teaspoon black pepper

Steps:

1. In a medium saucepan, melt the butter over medium heat. Add the garlic and thoroughly combine.

2. Add the cream cheese and whisk constantly until the cheese is melted. Slowly pour in the half-and-half and whisk continuously until smooth.

3. Gradually add the grated Parmesan, while whisking until combined.

4. Add the oregano, salt, and pepper, and stir. Continue to simmer for 1 to 2 minutes, but do not let the sauce boil. Add more salt and pepper, to taste, if desired.

5. Remove from the heat and serve, or refrigerate in airtight containers for up to 5 days.

Ranch Dressing

Makes 2 cups

Ingredients:

1 cup mayonnaise
½ cup sour cream
2 teaspoons lemon juice
2 teaspoons dried parsley
1 teaspoon dried dill
1 teaspoon dried chives
½ teaspoon garlic powder
½ teaspoon onion powder
½ teaspoon salt
½ teaspoon black pepper
¼ cup unsweetened
    almond milk

Steps:

1. Whisk all ingredients (except almond milk) until thoroughly combined.

2. Gradually whisk in the almond milk until the desired consistency has been reached.

3. Refrigerate for at least 1 hour and up to 10 days.

Low-Carb Pizza & Pasta Sauce

Makes 4 cups

Ingredients:

28 ounces peeled tomatoes
    (no sugar added)
1 tablespoon red wine
    vinegar
¼ cup olive oil
¼ teaspoon black pepper
½ teaspoon red pepper
    flakes
1 teaspoon onion powder
1 teaspoon garlic powder
1 teaspoon dried basil
1 teaspoon dried oregano
1 teaspoon dried parsley
Salt, to taste

Steps:

1. Puree the tomatoes, vinegar, olive oil, and ½ cup of the liquid from the can of tomatoes in a blender or food processor.

2. Stir in the remaining ingredients.

3. Taste and adjust seasoning as needed.

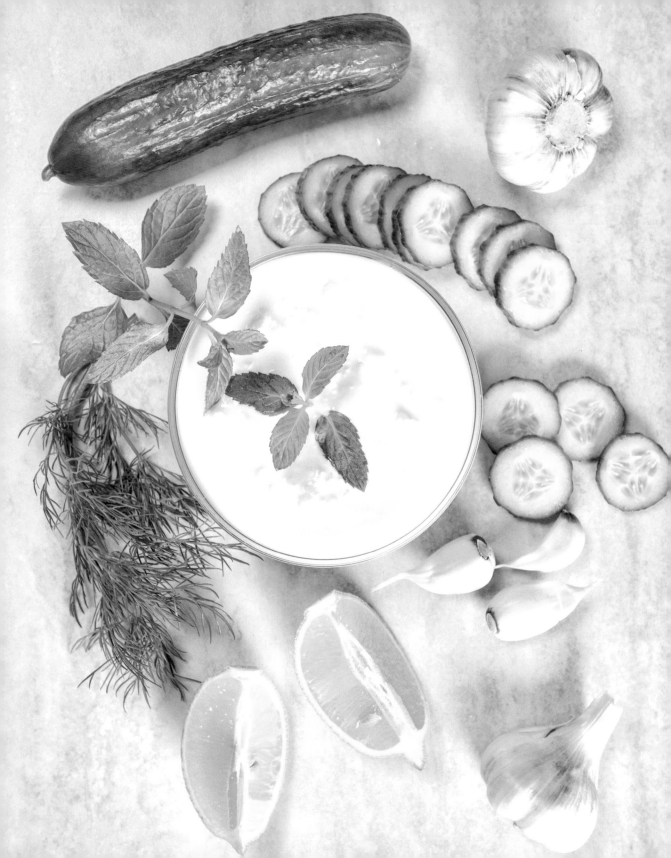

Tzatziki Dipping Sauce

Makes 1½ cups

Ingredients:

1 cup Greek whole milk
   yogurt
1 small cucumber, diced
2 cloves garlic, minced
2 tablespoons fresh lemon
   juice
2 tablespoons fresh dill,
   chopped
1 tablespoon fresh mint,
   finely chopped
Salt and pepper to taste
   (optional)

Steps:

1. In a medium mixing bowl combine all ingredients.

2. Store an in airtight container and refrigerate for up to 7 days.

Gorgonzola Sauce

Makes 1 cup

Ingredients:

1 clove garlic, minced
2 tablespoons butter
⅓ cup crumbled
   Gorgonzola cheese
¼ cup grated Parmesan
   cheese
¼ cup heavy cream
1 teaspoon onion powder
Salt and pepper, to taste

Steps:

1. In small saucepan over low heat, combine the garlic and butter.

2. When the butter is melted, add the remaining ingredients, stir, and raise the heat to medium-high.

3. Allow the sauce to come to a simmer and continue to stir for 3 to 5 minutes, allowing it to reduce until the desired consistency is achieved.

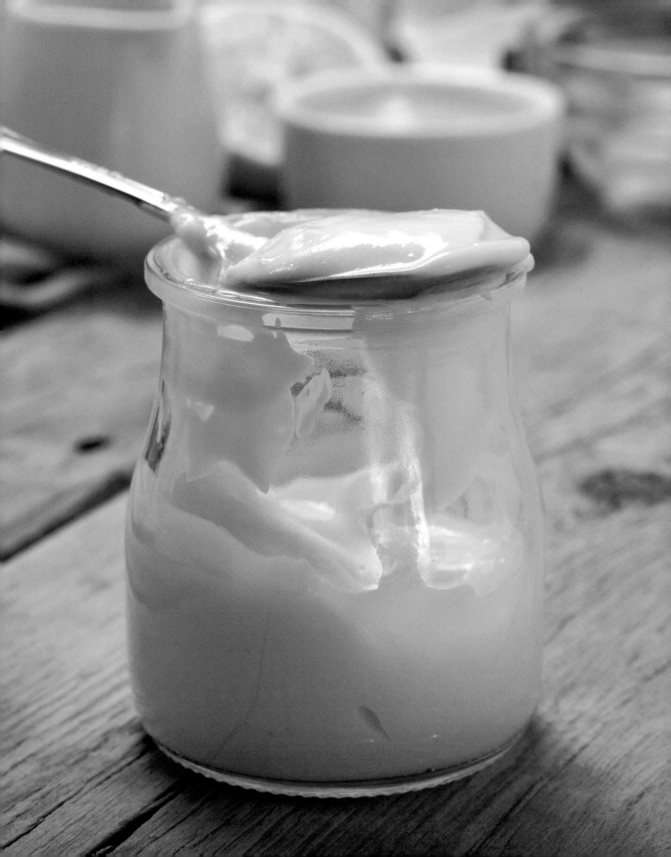

Avocado Oil Mayonnaise

Makes 1¼ cups

Ingredients:

1 large egg, at room temperature

1 teaspoon Dijon mustard

2 teaspoons apple cider vinegar

¼ teaspoon salt

1 cup avocado oil

Steps:

1. Crack the egg in a medium bowl and place all other ingredients on top.

2. Using a hand mixer, blend on medium-high heat until a mayonnaise texture forms.

3. Place in an airtight container and store in the refrigerator for up to 2 weeks.

Dairy-Free Cashew Cheese Sauce

Makes 2 cups

Ingredients:

1½ cups raw cashew pieces

¼ cup nutritional yeast flakes

1 teaspoon salt

¼ teaspoon garlic powder

3 tablespoons freshly squeezed lemon juice

¾ cup water

Steps:

1. In a food processor or blender, process the cashews into a fine powder, adding a drizzle of water if needed.

2. Add nutritional yeast, salt, and garlic powder, and process to combine.

3. Add lemon juice and water, and process until smooth.

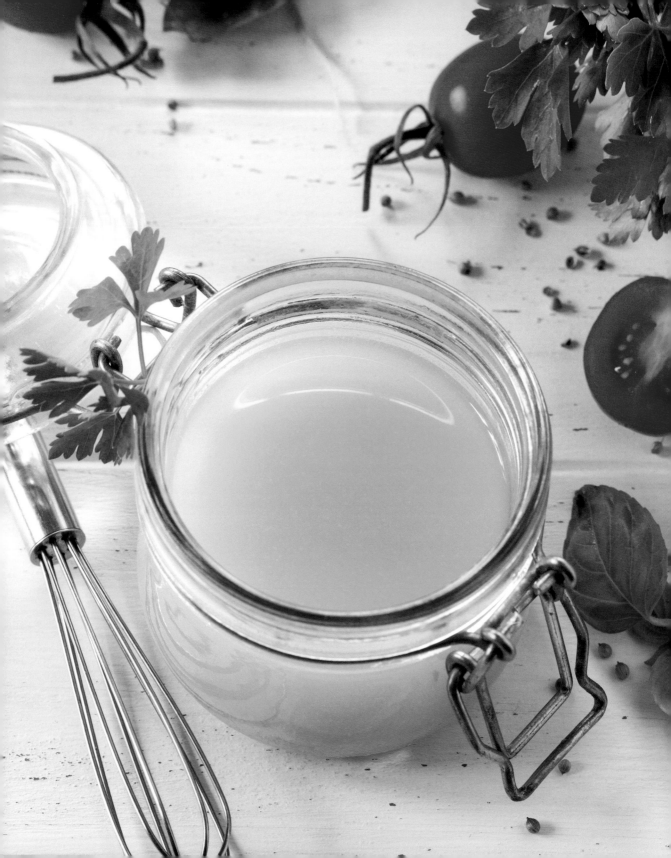

Lemon Vinaigrette

Makes 1 cup

Ingredients:

¼ cup red wine vinegar
2 tablespoons Dijon mustard
1 garlic clove, minced
1 teaspoon dried oregano
¼ teaspoon ground black pepper
½ cup olive oil
2 tablespoons fresh lemon juice

Steps:

1. Whisk red wine vinegar, mustard, garlic, oregano, and black pepper in a small bowl until blended.

2. Drizzle in oil, whisking until blended.

3. Beat lemon juice into the mixture.

Smooth Tomato and Goat Cheese Vinaigrette

Makes 1 cup

Ingredients:

¼ cup crumbled goat cheese
2 tablespoons white-wine vinegar
¼ cup extra-virgin olive oil
2 plum tomatoes, seeded and chopped
½ teaspoon salt
Freshly ground pepper, to taste
1 tablespoon chopped fresh tarragon (optional)

Steps:

1. Blend all ingredients together until mixture is creamy and smooth. This can be refrigerated for up to 3 days.

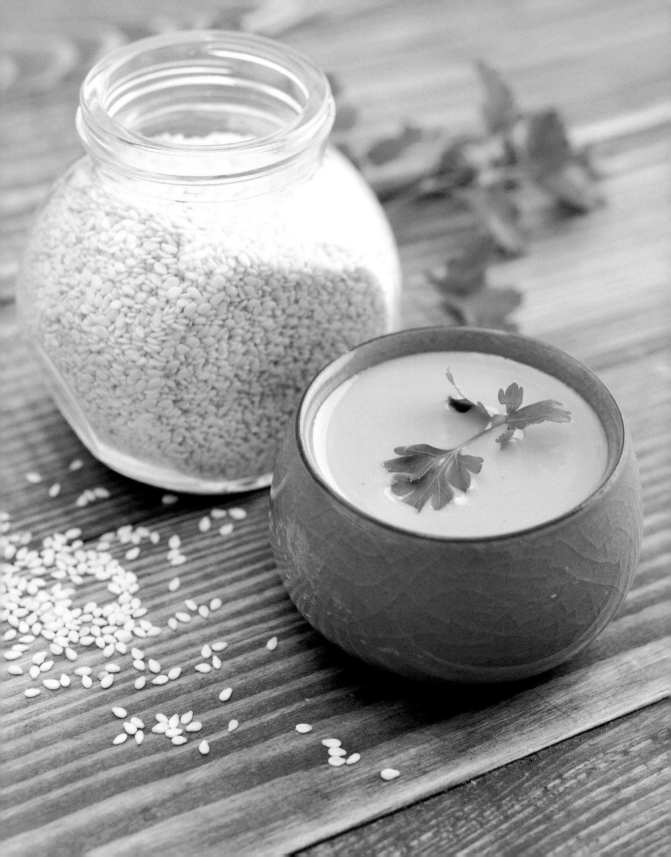

Creamy Tahini-Lemon Dressing

Makes 1 cup

Ingredients:

½ cup tahini
2 garlic cloves, minced
4 tablespoons fresh lemon
    juice
1 tablespoon extra-virgin
    olive oil
⅓ cup water
Salt and pepper, to taste

Steps:

1. Thoroughly combine all ingredients; add more water if needed until desired consistency is reached.

2. Store in the refrigerator in an airtight container for up to 7 days.

Easy Caesar Dressing

Makes 1 cup

Ingredients:

¾ cup mayonnaise
⅓ cup grated Parmesan
    cheese
2 garlic cloves, minced
1 teaspoon anchovy paste
1 teaspoon lemon juice
½ teaspoon Dijon mustard
Salt and pepper, to taste

Steps:

1. Place all ingredients in a medium-sized bowl and thoroughly combine.

2. Serve immediately or store in an airtight container in the refrigerator for up to 1 week.

Creamy Cucumber Vinaigrette

Makes 2 cups

Ingredients:

1 small cucumber, peeled, seeded, and chopped

¼ cup extra-virgin olive oil

2 tablespoons red wine vinegar

2 tablespoons chopped fresh chives

2 tablespoons chopped fresh parsley

2 tablespoons Greek yogurt

1 teaspoon prepared horseradish (optional)

Steps:

1. Blend all ingredients together until mixture is creamy and smooth.

Green Pesto

Makes 2 cups

Ingredients:

1½ cups fresh basil leaves (packed)

¼ teaspoon freshly ground black pepper

¼ cup freshly grated Parmigiano-Reggiano (optional)

2 tablespoons pine nuts or walnuts

1 teaspoon minced garlic

½ cup extra-virgin olive oil

Steps:

1. Using a food processor or blender, combine the basil and pepper and process/blend for a few seconds until the basil is chopped.

2. Add the cheese, pine nuts, and garlic and while the processor is running, add the oil in a thin, steady stream until you have reached a smooth consistency.

Horseradish Cream Sauce

Makes 1½ cups

Ingredients:

1 cup Greek yogurt

¼ cup grated fresh horseradish

1 tablespoon Dijon mustard

1 teaspoon white wine vinegar

¼ teaspoon freshly ground black pepper

Steps:

1. Place all ingredients into a medium mixing bowl and whisk until the mixture is smooth and creamy.

2. Refrigerate for at least 4 hours to allow flavors to meld.

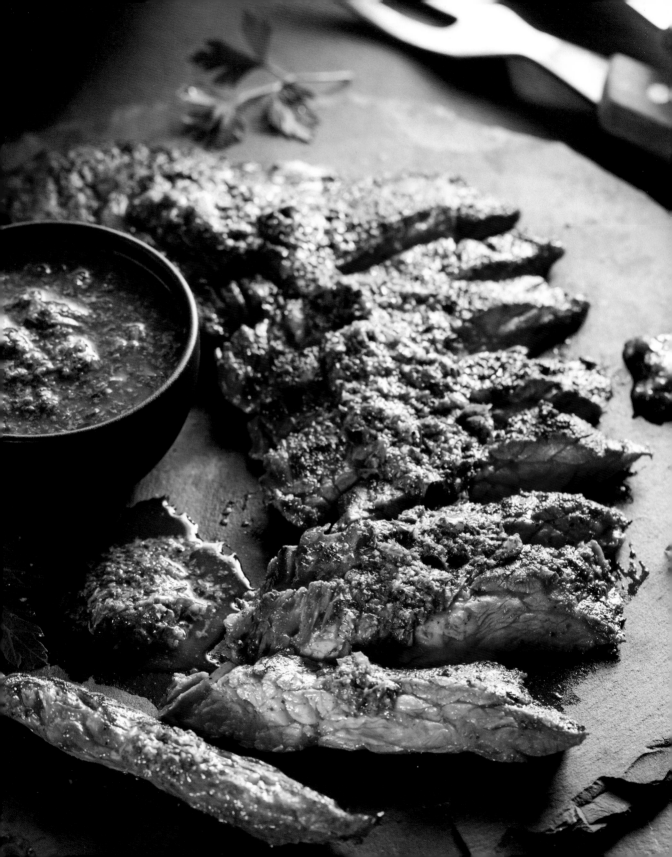

Chimichurri Sauce

Makes 1 cup

Ingredients:

1 bunch parsley, finely
   chopped
1 bunch cilantro, finely
   chopped
3 tablespoons capers, finely
   chopped
2 garlic cloves, minced
1½ tablespoons red wine
   vinegar
½ teaspoon red pepper
   flakes
½ teaspoon ground black
   pepper
½ cup extra-virgin olive oil

Steps:

1. Put the parsley, cilantro, capers, and garlic in a medium
   mixing bowl and toss to combine.

2. Add the vinegar, red and black pepper, and stir.

3. Pour in the olive oil and mix until well combined; let sit
   for 30 minutes so that the flavors blend.

White Wine Sauce

Makes 1 cup

Ingredients:

½ cup chicken broth
¼ cup white wine
Juice of ½ lemon
1 tablespoon minced
   shallot
1 garlic clove, minced
1 tablespoon butter
1 tablespoon extra-virgin
   olive oil
Black pepper, to taste

Steps:

1. Combine all ingredients in pan and use as a simmer
   sauce.

Cooking Measurements Conversion Charts

US Dry Volume Measurements

MEASURE	EQUIVALENT
⅟₁₆ teaspoon	Dash
⅛ teaspoon	Pinch
3 teaspoons	1 Tablespoon
⅛ cup	2 Tablespoons (= 1 standard coffee scoop)
⅛ cup	4 Tablespoons
⅛ cup	5 Tablespoons plus 1 teaspoon
½ cup	8 Tablespoons
¾ cup	12 Tablespoons
1 cup	16 Tablespoons
1 Pound	16 Ounces (oz.)

US to Metric Conversions

⅕ teaspoon	1 milliliter (ml)
1 teaspoon	5 ml
1 tablespoon	15 ml
1 fluid oz.	30 ml
⅕ cup	50 ml
1 cup	240 ml
2 cups (1 pint)	470 ml
4 cups (1 quart)	.95 liter
4 quarts (1 gal.)	3.8 liters
1 oz.	28 grams
1 pound	454 grams

US Liquid Volume Measurements

8 Fluid ounces	1 Cup
1 Pint	2 Cups (= 16 fluid ounces)
1 Quart	2 Pints (= 4 cups)
1 Gallon	4 Quarts (= 16 cups)

Metric to US Conversions

1 milliliter (ml)	⅕ teaspoon
5 ml	1 teaspoon
15 ml	1 tablespoon
30 ml	1 fluid oz.
100 ml	3.4 fluid oz.
240 ml	1 cup
1 liter	34 fluid oz.
1 liter	4.2 cups
1 liter	2.1 pints
1 liter	1.06 quarts
1 liter	.26 gallon
1 gram	.035 ounce
100 grams	3.5 ounces
500 grams	1.10 pounds
1 kilogram	2.205 pounds
1 kilogram	35 oz.

Oven Temperature Conversions	
FAHRENHEIT	**CELSIUS**
275º F	140º C
300º F	150º C
325º F	165º C
350º F	180º C
375º F	190º C
400º F	200º C
425º F	220º C
450º F	230º C
475º F	240º C

Measures for Pans and Dishes	
INCHES	**CENTIMETERS**
9-by-13-inch baking dish	22-by-33-centimeter baking dish
8-by-8-inch baking dish	20-by-20-centimeter baking dish
9-by-5-inch loaf pan (8 cups in capacity)	23-by-12-centimeter loaf pan (2 liters in capacity)

CALORIES	KILOJOULES
1	4.1868
1,500	6,276
1,600	6,694
1,700	7,113
1,800	7,531
1,900	7,950
2,000	8,368
2,100	8,786
2,200	9,205
2,300	9,623
2,400	10,042
2,500	10,460

Acknowledgments

This book was written during a very challenging time for the world. We would like to thank every single healthcare professional and essential worker who sacrificed to get us through. Thank you from the bottom of our hearts.

About the Authors

Aimee Aristotelous, author of *Almost Keto* and *The Whole Pregnancy*, is a certified nutritionist, specializing in ketogenic and gluten-free nutrition, as well as prenatal dietetics. She is a contributor for a variety of publications including *Health, People, HuffPost*, Parade, Yahoo! News, INSIDER, Motherly, *Consumer Health Digest, Simply Gluten-Free, Well + Good*, National Celiac Association, and *Delight Gluten-Free*. She has appeared on the morning show in Los Angeles as a regular speaker for the nationwide Nourished Festival, and has been the exclusive nutritionist for NBC affiliate KSEE 24 News in California, appearing in more than fifty nutrition and cooking segments. Aimee has nine years of nutrition consulting experience and has helped over 3,000 people lose weight and get healthy!

Aimee's interest in nutrition began as she struggled with her own high cholesterol and weight gain after taking a sedentary office job in her twenties, once her athletic career came to an end. She furthered her nutrition education in the ketogenic and gluten-free realms after applying those dietary lifestyles to resolve her bad cholesterol, weight gain, and other dietary-related ailments such as migraine headaches. In addition to her Nutrition and Wellness certification through American Fitness Professionals and Associates, Aimee has a bachelor's degree in business/marketing from California State University, Long Beach. A California native, she currently resides in Fort Lauderdale, Florida, with her husband, Richard, and son, Alex, and enjoys the beach, cooking, and traveling.

Richard Oliva, author of *Almost Keto*, is a certified nutritionist who specializes in ketogenic, gluten-free, and sports nutrition. He is a third-degree black belt in judo who has competed internationally and won state, national, and international titles. He has conducted numerous nutrition seminars for colleges, health clubs, and medical practices, and has appeared in numerous nutrition and cooking segments on NBC affiliate KSEE 24 News in California. He loves to share his lifetime passion for both nutrition and judo and has helped thousands of people learn how to eat better and improve their health and fitness.

Richard began studying nutrition at about the same time that he started learning judo in the mid-1970s, when he was in high school. He became a passionate student of nutrition after one of his coworkers told him, "You know, you're killing yourself!" as Richard was eating a donut and drinking a soda during his break. That comment launched him on a mission to learn everything he could about nutrition and health.

Richard earned his Nutrition and Wellness certification through American Fitness Professionals and Associates. He also has a Bachelor of Science degree in geology from Kent State University in Kent, Ohio. An Ohio native, he currently resides in Fort Lauderdale, Florida, with Aimee and Alex. Richard still enjoys practicing judo as well as weight training, cooking, and traveling.

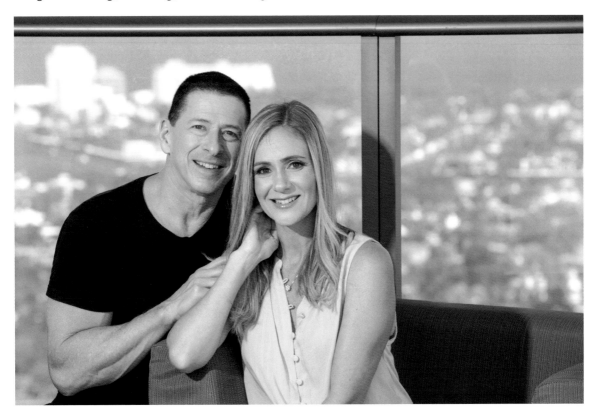

References

Avena, N., P. Rada, and B. Hoebel. "Evidence for Sugar Addiction: Behavioral and Neurochemical Effects of Intermittent, Excessive Sugar Intake." NCBI. Neuroscience and Biobehavioral Reviews, January 2008. ncbi.nlm.nih.gov/pmc/articles/PMC2235907/.

Callegaro, D., and J. Tirapegui. "[Comparison of the Nutritional Value between Brown Rice and White Rice]." NCBI. October/November 1996. Accessed April 14, 2019. https://www.ncbi.nlm.nih.gov/pubmed /9302338.

Chinwong, S., D. Chinwong, and A. Mangklabruks. "Daily Consumption of Virgin Coconut Oil Increases High-Density Lipoprotein Cholesterol Levels in Healthy Volunteers: A Randomized Crossover Trial." NCBI. December 14, 2017. Accessed May 19, 2019. https://www.ncbi.nlm.nih.gov/pmc/articles/PMC5745680/.

Damle, S. G. "Smart Sugar? The Sugar Conspiracy." NCBI. July 24, 2017. Accessed March 7, 2019. https: //www.ncbi.nlm.nih.gov/pmc/articles/PMC5551319/.

Dewan, S. "Global Markets for Sugars and Sweeteners in Processed Foods and Beverages." BCC Research, June 2015.

"Diet Review: Ketogenic Diet for Weight Loss." The Nutrition Source, May 22, 2019. hsph.harvard.edu /nutritionsource/healthy-weight/diet-reviews/ketogenic-diet/.

Feskanich et al., "Milk, dietary calcium, and bone fractures in women: a 12-year prospective study.," NCBI, June 1997, accessed September 11, 2017. ncbi.nlm.nih.gov/pmc/articles/PMC1380936/.

"Food Waste in America in 2020: Statistics & Facts: RTS," accessed June 10, 2020. rts.com/resources /guides/food-waste-america/.

Gostin, Lawrence O. ""Big Food" Is Making America Sick." NCBI. September 13, 2013. Accessed March 7, 2019. ncbi.nlm.nih.gov/pmc/articles/PMC5020160/

Kaats, G. R., D. Bagchi, and H. G. Preuss. "Konjac Glucomannan Dietary Supplementation Causes Significant Fat Loss in Compliant Overweight Adults." NCBI. October 22, 2015. Accessed May 20, 2019. ncbi.nlm.nih.gov/pubmed/26492494.

Kabara, J., D. Swieczkowski, A. Conley, and J. Truant. "Fatty Acids and Derivatives as Antimicrobial Agents." NCBI. July 1972. Accessed May 19, 2019. ncbi.nlm.nih.gov/pmc/articles/PMC444260/.

Koller, VJ, M. Furhacker, A. Nersesyan, M. Misik, M. Eisenbauer, and S. Knasmueller. "Cytotoxic and DNA-damaging Properties of Glyphosate and Roundup in Human-derived Buccal Epithelial Cells." NCBI. May 2012. Accessed May 11, 2019. ncbi.nlm.nih.gov/pubmed/22331240.

Malekinejad and A. Rezabakhsh, "Hormones in Dairy Foods and Their Impact on Public Health—A Narrative Review Article," June 2015, accessed September 10, 2017. ncbi.nlm.nih.gov/pmc/articles/PMC4524299/.

Maruyama, T. Oshima, and K. Ohyama, "Exposure to exogenous estrogen through intake of commercial milk produced from pregnant cows.," NCBI, February 2010, accessed September 20, 2017. ncbi.nlm.nih.gov/pubmed/19496976.

McNamara, Donald. "The Fifty Year Rehabilitation of the Egg." NCBI. October 2015. Accessed April 27, 2019. ncbi.nlm.nih.gov/pmc/articles/PMC4632449/.

Michaëlsson, K. et al., "Milk intake and risk of mortality and fractures in women and men: cohort studies.," NCBI, October 28, 2014, accessed September 20, 2017. ncbi.nlm.nih.gov/pubmed/25352269.

Micsmeanderings, M., Evan Lavizadeh, Alireza, Bryan A Matsumoto, Marco, Emily, et al. "Natural and Added Sugars: Two Sides of the Same Coin," October 5, 2015. sitn.hms.harvard.edu/flash/2015/natural-and-added-sugars-two-sides-of-the-same-coin/.

Missimer, A., D. DiMarco, C. Andersen, A. Murillo, M. Vergara-Jiminez, and M. Fernandez. "Consuming Two Eggs per Day, as Compared to an Oatmeal Breakfast, Decreases Plasma Ghrelin While Maintaining the LDL/HDL Ratio." NCBI. February 01, 2017. Accessed April 27, 2019. ncbi.nlm.nih.gov/pmc/articles/PMC5331520/.

Mozaffarian, Dariush, Tao Hao, Eric Rimm, Walter Willett, and Frank Hu. "Changes in Diet and Lifestyle and Long-Term Weight Gain in Women and Men." The New England Journal of Medicine. June 29, 2011. Accessed April 14, 2019. nejm.org/doi/full/10.1056/NEJMoa1014296.

Mumme, K., and W. Stonehouse. "Effects of Medium-chain Triglycerides on Weight Loss and Body Composition: A Meta-analysis of Randomized Controlled Trials." NCBI. February 2015. Accessed May 19, 2019. ncbi.nlm.nih.gov/pubmed/25636220.

Nestle, M. "Food Lobbies, the Food Pyramid, and U.S. Nutrition Policy." NCBI. July 1, 1993. Accessed February 16, 2019. ncbi.nlm.nih.gov/pubmed/8375951.

Ng, S. W., M. M. Slining, and B. M. Popkin. (2012). Use of caloric and noncaloric sweeteners in US consumer packaged foods, 2005–2009. Journal of the Academy of Nutrition and Dietetics, 112(11), 1828–1834. e1821-1826.

Niaz, K., E. Zaplatic, and J. Spoor. "Extensive Use of Monosodium Glutamate: A Threat to Public Health?" NCBI. March 19, 2018. Accessed May 11, 2019. ncbi.nlm.nih.gov/pmc/articles/PMC5938543/.

Paoli, Antonio. "Ketogenic Diet for Obesity: Friend or Foe?" NCBI. February 01, 2014. Accessed March 23, 2019. ncbi.nlm.nih.gov/pmc/articles/PMC3945587/.

C. S. Pase et al., "Influence of perinatal trans fat on behavioral responses and brain oxidative status of adolescent rats acutely exposed to stress.," NCBI, September 5, 2013, accessed September 2, 2017. ncbi.nlm.nih.gov/pubmed/23742847.

Samsel, A., and S. Seneff. "Glyphosate, Pathways to Modern Diseases II: Celiac Sprue and Gluten Intolerance." NCBI. December 2013. Accessed May 11, 2019. ncbi.nlm.nih.gov/pmc/articles/PMC3945755/.

Santarelli, R. L., F. Pierre, and D. Corpet. "Processed Meat and Colorectal Cancer: A Review of Epidemiologic and Experimental Evidence." NCBI. March 25, 2008. Accessed April 14, 2019. ncbi.nlm.nih.gov/pmc/articles/PMC2661797/.

Soffritti, M., M. Padovani, E. Tibaldi, L. Falcioni, F. Manservisi, and F. Belpoggi. "The Carcinogenic Effects of Aspartame: The Urgent Need for Regulatory Re-evaluation." NCBI. April 2014. Accessed April 14, 2019. ncbi.nlm.nih.gov/pubmed/24436139.

Spero, David. "Is Milk Bad for You? Diabetes and Milk - Diabetes Self." Management. Diabetes Self Management, June 20, 2017. diabetesselfmanagement.com/blog/is-milk-bad-for-you-diabetes-and-milk/.

Stockman, Mary-Catherine et al., "Intermittent Fasting: Is the Wait Worth the Weight?," June 2018. ncbi.nlm.nih.gov/pmc/articles/PMC5959807/.

"Sugar & The Diet." The Sugar Association. Accessed March 5, 2020. sugar.org/diet/.

Swithers, S. "Artificial sweeteners produce the counterintuitive effect of inducing metabolic derangements," NCBI, September 2013, accessed September 24, 2017. ncbi.nlm.nih.gov/pmc/articles/PMC3772345/.

Zhang, G., A. Pan, G. Zhong, Z. Yu, H. Wu, X. Chen, L. Tang, Y. Feng, H. Zhou, H. Li, B. Hong, W. C. Willett, V. S. Malik, D. Spiegelman, F. B. Hu, and X. Lin. "Substituting White Rice with Brown Rice for 16 Weeks Does Not Substantially Affect Metabolic Risk Factors in Middle-aged Chinese Men and Women with Diabetes or a High Risk for Diabetes." NCBI. September 01, 2011. Accessed April 14, 2019. ncbi.nlm.nih.gov/pubmed/21795429.

Index